Never
Simple

For Judith Scheier, who tried.

Never Simple

Liz Scheier

HENRY HOLT AND COMPANY
NEW YORK

Henry Holt and Company
Publishers since 1866
120 Broadway
New York, NY 10271
www.henryholt.com

Henry Holt ® and Ⓗ® are registered trademarks of Macmillan
Publishing Group, LLC.

Library of Congress Cataloging-in-Publication Data

Names: Scheier, Liz, author.
Title: Never simple : a memoir / Liz Scheier.
Description: First edition. | New York : Henry Holt and Company,
    2022.
Identifiers: LCCN 2021019083 (print) | LCCN 2021019084
    (ebook) | ISBN 9781250823137 (hardcover) |
    ISBN 9781250823120 (ebook)
Subjects: LCSH: Scheier, Liz. | Mental illness—United States—
    Biography. | Mentally ill parents—United States—Biography. |
    Mothers and daughters—United States.
Classification: LCC RC463 .S34 2022 (print) | LCC RC463 (ebook) |
    DDC 616.890092 [B]—dc23
LC record available at https://lccn.loc.gov/2021019083
LC ebook record available at https://lccn.loc.gov/2021019084

Our books may be purchased in bulk for promotional, educational,
or business use. Please contact your local bookseller or the
Macmillan Corporate and Premium Sales Department at
(800) 221-7945, extension 5442, or by e-mail at
MacmillanSpecialMarkets@macmillan.com.

The names and identifying details of some persons described in this
book have been changed.

First Edition 2022

Designed by Meryl Sussman Levavi

Printed in the United States of America

10 9 8 7 6 5 4 3 2 1

The truth is rarely pure and never simple.

—Oscar Wilde

He who tells a lie is not sensible of how great a task he undertakes; for he must be forced to invent twenty more to maintain that one.

—Alexander Pope

When we discover that someone we trusted can be trusted no longer, it forces us to reexamine the universe, to question the whole instinct and concept of trust. For a while, we are thrust back onto some bleak, jutting ledge, in a dark pierced by sheets of fire, swept by sheets of rain, in a world before kinship, or naming, or tenderness exist; we are brought close to formlessness.

—Adrienne Rich

Contents

Liars

"I need to tell you something."

I looked up over the edge of my book. My mother was standing in the living room doorway in one of her endless array of flowered, crepey muumuus—the Shut-In Chic Collection, I called them privately—with one hand on the knob, her face grave. I was on fall break, my freshman year at college; the last year, after this conversation, that I would consider my mother's apartment home. I let the book fall facedown on my chest.

"What?"

"Well." She fiddled with the knob, coughed. "You said you were going to take driving lessons and get a learner's permit when you go back to school."

"That's right."

"That's going to be . . . hard. I don't think they'll give you one."

I laughed, a little offended. "I'm sure it can't be *that* hard. Millions of idiots do it every day."

"That's not what I mean. *Look*." More fiddling. "They're going to ask you for identification, a birth certificate. You don't have one."

"So I'll send away for a copy."

"No. No. Will you *listen* to what I'm saying? There's nothing to get a copy of. I never filed a record of your birth at all."

I scrabbled my elbows under me and sat up, my breath sharp in my throat. *Finally*, I thought. *This is it*. A bureaucratic boulder she couldn't lie her way over. An official document even she wouldn't dare forge. At last: answers. "I don't understand. Why not?"

"Well." Deep breath. "I was married when you were born. But not to your father."

❖ ❖ ❖

No one lies like family.

We lie to each other all the time. We lie to keep each other at a distance, to give ourselves some elbow room in the claustrophobic nuclear unit. To spare each other's feelings. To cut short a conversation, or to begin one. To ensure that the artichoke-heart softness of our insides is sealed safely off forever. As I write this, my two toddlers are in the next room, cheerfully belting out some interminable preschool song and throwing stuffed animals at each other. They're too young to ask me about my missing father, or my never-spoken-of mother, or why I am the way I am. They're too young to understand how much they don't know.

Then again, I haven't started lying to them. Yet.

This is the story of digging out the biggest lie I was ever told.

Never
Simple

CHAPTER I

The Man Who Wasn't There

My father was long since dead, but never mind: we had each other. My stylish, petite, sardonic mother and me. There weren't a lot of single mothers around, and the few we knew—heads together in the playground, Marlboro Reds gesturing furiously, given a wide berth by the married women sheep-dogging their husbands away—were divorced. Mom was a widow, without any of the usual indicators that archaic, weepy word implies—no black dresses, no red-rimmed eyes. He was too long gone for that. He was forgotten. We were a team: one big, one small. Two sparrow-boned, sharp-eyed blondes, hand in hand.

There was no trace of my dead father except an ancient white leather backgammon set, which I kept reverently boxed up under my bed. She'd married him not long after divorcing her first husband, and in the early weeks of her pregnancy, he was killed in a car accident when he stopped at a red light and the driver behind him didn't. In a storm of grief she burned all his photos, including those from their wedding, at which she wore a borrowed ivory pantsuit that she dutifully returned. It was such a whirlwind romance that even the few friends she didn't alienate—and the very few members of our family who were alive and speaking to each other—had never met him. Family, dead. Friends, moved away.

This story is, of course, total bullshit.

But I believed it. Why wouldn't I? Parents in children's books died all the time. I was a city kid, and as far as I was concerned, cars—in which I almost never rode—were gas-snorting, two-ton death machines.

I asked about him, anxious for the details.

"What did he look like?"

"Like you, Miss Mouse. Blond, gorgeous." (I blushed.)

"Was he excited to have me?"

"It was too early, honey. He didn't know."

"Oh." That stumped me, the specifics of pregnancy fuzzy at best. Then: "What was he *like*?"

She pushed up her glasses into her hair and sighed. "Elizabeth, this was all a long time ago. He was a good man. I'm sorry he's gone, but he's gone. Now, what should we read tonight?"

I worshipped her. I loved her smoky cackle and her jokes, even though most of them went over my head, and I loved her whole-body storytelling, and her habit of pulling me out of school whenever something more interesting was happening. I loved that she adored me above everything else on earth and told me so on a roughly hourly basis. I felt like the small, slightly ratty sun around which the galaxy revolved.

So how was it possible that she was lying to me?

The paucity of belongings wasn't the problem. I could

believe that a person could be swept away wholesale with nothing to show he was ever there. But the stories were such clear fabrications, haltingly told, a note of panic in her voice. She wasn't a good liar, despite all the practice.

The other kids I knew who were missing a father hadn't misplaced theirs quite so badly. Theirs came to pick them up for brunch on Sunday mornings, or dinner every other Thursday. They may have been shitty, and plenty of them were, but they were known quantities. Mine was a blank with a fuzzy blond halo and, apparently, a love for backgammon. Was he out there somewhere—in a Kips Bay divorced-guy apartment, or a row house in Queens—wondering if she'd ever let him meet me? Or unaware I existed at all? I surreptitiously scanned the faces of blond men on the street who looked to be about the right age. *Is it you?* Years later, when I donated eggs, I did the same with tiny blond toddlers with a mixture of curiosity and detachment. My anonymous genetic children were hypotheticals, but my father—he had to have been real. (Evidence: me.) But where was he?

Telling exorbitant lies was easier in the 80s. There was no internet, no way to track down the clues, especially for a six-year-old who rarely left the house. ("If any of your friends' fathers touch you, *you tell me*," she warned, even though she usually insisted playdates take place in our own living room, under her watchful eye.) She could reasonably believe that if she didn't give up the truth, I would never find out. But I knew something was wrong with her story. She was reluctant to talk about him, and I suspected that her reticence wasn't due to the patina of grief, but the fear of slipping up. What was she hiding?

The obvious answer, to me, was that he was still alive.

When I was very young, I thought: A spy! An astronaut abandoned on a distant planet! The foreign service! Wrongfully
imprisoned in a case of mistaken identity! Older and more
cynical, I thought: married.

I knew perfectly well that there was a lie happening, somewhere, but I couldn't parse out to whom it had been told.

I did have his name: Warren Steven Livingston. I repeated
it to myself, turning it over and over in my mind. I printed
it in careful capitals on the Hebrew school submission forms
for trees planted in Israel in the name of a loved one in
exchange for donations to the Jewish National Fund. I hung
the certificates proudly on the wall, and my mother winced
and averted her eyes every time she passed. One memorable
day while she left my eight-year-old self alone for an hour
while running errands, I called every Livingston in the New
York City white pages, trembling, asking if they were related
to him. No one was; their brusque voices softened when they
heard my high-pitched child's voice. But none of them knew
a Warren Steven.

It will not surprise you—you will probably already have
figured out—that no one recognized the name because she made
it up. When she finally admitted the lie, that day in the living
room, she told me she was afraid I would find the place where
he'd died—a stretch of sidewalk only two blocks away from
my childhood home—and make a shrine out of it. I'm skeptical. I think the real reason is that she was putting off the day I
would find out her two shames: that he wasn't Jewish, and that
they weren't married. Well: not to each other, anyway.

I speed-rifled through her room, paging through old
photo albums, while she was down in our apartment building's hot, airless laundry room. Somewhere, there had to be

clues as to the story that was more and more evidently untrue. But my career as a pint-sized secret agent was short-lived and unsuccessful—her filing cabinet was locked tight, and I never could find where she hid the key—and I tried hard to forget about the man who wasn't there. She must have a good reason, I thought. Anyone can learn to live with a lie.

And so: there we were. Mother and daughter. Senior and junior. A comedy act, a vaudeville team. But I had no idea who I was really living with, only that she transformed behind that locked apartment door.

CHAPTER 2

Yorkville on My Mind

Think of New York City in the 70s and 80s and you think: Blackout, riots. Tagged subway cars and a pre-Giuliani Times Square, lined with head shops and hookers. Crime and needles and the concrete jungle. But it was also a time when you could live on a regular income in Manhattan, could take kids' art classes at the Metropolitan Museum for next to nothing, and get $20 rush tickets to Broadway shows. My New York was Shirley Temples in tiki mugs at Panda Garden on Second Avenue, old Hungarian men patting my hair as I raced past the Orthodox church on Seventy-Ninth Street, Simon & Garfunkel's concert in Central Park, a picnic blanket and a battered Pan Am carrier bag full of sandwiches, wine for her and milk for me. The tree at Rockefeller Center, sure, but also the origami tree at the Museum of Natural History, where volunteers fashioned fiddler crabs and the Empire State Building out of shiny paper.

I was born in Yorkville, the very far east of Manhattan's Upper East Side, which butts up against the gray-green East River. This was not the Upper East Side of mansions and embassies, Park Avenue duplexes and the Metropolitan Museum. Yorkville had been heavily settled by German immigrants, and the briny smell of the East River mixed with the meaty, spicy scent of sausages wafting out of Schaller and Weber is the olfactory record of my childhood. Let Proust have his prim, delicate madeleines; I'll take the salty bite of bratwurst any day.

Jews name their babies after dead relatives, for reasons both superstitious and practical. If a child is named after a living older person, we reason, the Angel of Death, apparently both nearsighted and not particularly bright, may sweep up the baby when it's the grandmother's time. Reserving the name-honor for the dead also keeps the family peace. No one's fighting over who gets a baby named after them when naming after the living is bad luck.

Mom took that one step further and named me after Queen Elizabeth I, to whom we were definitely not related. She didn't bother to name me at all for the first six months; I was born at home, and it's not like there was anyone else around who could credibly be confused with "the baby." When she finally did, she hit me with the one-two punch of Verity as a middle name. "I was considering Verity, Chastity, and Serenity," she said to a friend, airily. "But then I figured I wouldn't wish chastity on her, and no child of mine is going to be serene." (I dined out on that one for *years*.)

Verity, from the Latin "veritas," meaning truth. What's in a name? Probably nothing. But for all my faults, I am very truthful.

Like most New Yorkers, we lived in a space most outsiders would consider outrageously small, but which was plenty for us. The one-bedroom apartment had a large closet in the entry hall that had been converted to accommodate a twin bed for my mother, and I lived in the bedroom. That apartment now probably costs the earth, but in the 80s Yorkville was a quiet, middle-class grid of beneficently wide avenues and brownstoned cross streets. We lived just above an Associated, a grocery chain that carried enough kosher food to assuage the conscience during Passover and enough bacon to calm the soul the rest of the year.

Mom didn't work, or didn't work anymore—she had "retired" in her late thirties from her career as an attorney specializing in copyright protections—and I didn't know enough to understand that this was strange. She hired a middle-aged woman named Margaret, a recent immigrant from Hungary, to care for me and run our lives, keeping my kid clutter in check and carefully forking sputtering, golden hand-cut French fries from pans of oil for Hanukkah parties and birthdays. Margaret had a nervous poodle named Pepper and a handsome, reticent husband, Sandor; he took me to Father's Day dances at their church and swung me through the steps, his gleaming shoes tapping and my braids flying.

We went to museums and to the ballet, to puppet shows in Central Park and ice-skating on Wollman Rink (I skating, my mother sitting on the rinkside bench with hot chocolate); only tourists went to the showy, expensive Rockefeller Center. I clambered over the rocks near Belvedere Castle and wandered in the Ramble, she sometimes speeding us up, talking loudly, to cover up the evidence of what I now know was the most active cruising ground of the carefree gay early 80s. We bought lychee from the street carts in Chinatown and giant brown-paper-wrapped multipacks of wintergreen Life Savers from Peter, the hot dog seller on the corner of Ninety-Sixth Street, just above the entrance to the C train, who was no more immune to her charms than any other man she met. "Have the most wonderful day, Mrs. Scheier!" he'd beam, handing over the carton, the rolls heavy like a box of ammunition. No one called her Judith. No one would dare.

We never took subways. No one I knew did; they roared through the tunnels on shrieking tracks, reeking of urine and so heavily tagged that you couldn't tell the original paint color. We walked most places or took Checker cabs, where I begged, as a treat, to sit on the seatbelt-less jump seats that folded down from the divider, which even the toughest-looking drivers slid shut, looking askance over their shoulders, as my mother chain-smoked in the back. We took lumbering cross-town buses that wheezed consumptively across the transverses, and the swifter M104 down Broadway to go to the theater.

On New Year's Eve we went to Zabar's and bought one of everything that looked good: babka, lox, pickled herring in cream sauce, tiny crisp cornichons and giant full-sour pickles. "Do we really need all this?" I'd ask, sagging under the weight of the bags. "Oh, reason not the need, child!" she Lear-quoted, and marched us across the street to H&H for bagels. She arranged it all carefully on bright primary-color trays, and we celebrated our annual Great American Pig-Out in front of the TV, watching the ball drop on Times Square

Every June, she threw a sumptuous birthday party; the year I turned six, on 6/6, she threw a whopping six. For my second birthday, all my tiny friends clambered on the gym equipment at the 92nd Street Y; for my eighth, we played with fossils and ate novelty dinosaur-shaped chicken tenders at the American Museum of Natural History. For my tenth, the Bronx Zoo, with handsome animal puppets, a different one for each child, from Toy City on Eighty-Sixth Street. I was her one shot, and by God, she was going to do it up right.

So: Where did the money come from?

How were we affording these parties, these presents? How were we going away for a month every summer? How were we paying the *mortgage*?

A mystery.

She wasn't a big fan of children's books, and so she read me classics starting when I was four—*The Yearling*, *A Tale of Two Cities*, *David Copperfield*. I lay next to her on the couch, my legs hooked over hers and head resting on her arm as she read aloud, pausing to take drags off the ever-present cigarette smoldering in her cut-glass ashtray. We kept a legal pad handy to note the words she couldn't define, rare though they were, to look up later, and gave up on the dense *Last of the Mohicans* when the list in her neat but illegible handwriting ran to a full page. Those few kids' books she did read me were heavily annotated to suit her sensibilities; I was an adult before I learned that Christopher Robin was not the only male character in the Winnie-the-Pooh books.

She still left the apartment in those days. She still had friends. She knew there was something not quite right about our home, although she thought it was the fact that she was a single mother. She constructed a village from scratch, providing half a dozen father figures, deliberately and carefully cultivated. Her friend Jim, an illustrator who sketched out Greek heroes and puppies at his giant drafting table as I sat spellbound in his lap; her friend Shannon's husband, a grave, Lincoln-bearded man who tried and failed to teach me to pitch; the wheelchair-bound Holocaust survivor down the hall. But they all belonged to someone else; they were someone else's daddy. I didn't want the shades-of-gray connection to a man who was only peripherally mine. I wanted the DNA connection, the guy who was mine and mine alone.

I craved a picture, desperately. If I couldn't smell his neck or hear his voice or feel the hoist of his arms from ground to hip, I wanted to know what his face looked like. I wanted a glimpse of the physical fact of him—the real person—even if what he really was was dead.

But I rarely said a word, as even the most off-handed question ended in tears, whether hers or mine or both. She'd claim ignorance and a poor memory—They had known each other for so short a time! It was so long ago!—and then retreat to her room, where she cried herself blotchy, emerging shiny eyed and edgy as a feral cat. I shut my mouth and kept it shut.

Her rage had a very specific smell, like the ozone sting that fills your nostrils when the anesthesiologist turns on the pump. I could pick up the smell of fury from across the room, and hear it in the slap of her slippers as she crossed the apartment. Slow was normal, fast was danger, and a half-run meant I'd better leap out of that bed and lock myself in the bathroom. Fast.

There was no telling what would set her off. It was never the same day to day. If an interaction didn't inspire irritation, it inspired rage, and if not rage, fits of weeping. When the building's handyman mistook my sled, set against the wall of the emergency stairwell to drip-dry, for garbage, she flew into a tantrum and screamed at him that he was too stupid to live.

A screed on the letterhead of the law firm for which she had once worked followed, and I never saw him again. I proudly showed her a dress I'd stitched for her childhood doll, and her eyes lit on a hairline crack on the doll's age-hardened rubber leg, the consequence of my six-year-old hands pulling the comically too-small dress over it. She fell prostrate on the bed, her face buried in the doll, in a rush of angry tears. "Oh *Bethy*," she wailed. "I'm so sorry. I'm so sorry. I didn't know she'd break you with her stupid dress!"

Leaving a water glass in the sink went unnoticed nine times out of ten, but the tenth time, lightning crackled through the air. She rarely hit me, but it was her voice I feared; her eyes glistened and sparked, and she screamed so loud, and with such abandon, that her eyes slid out of focus and spittle clung to her chin. It was the lack of control that was so terrifying. You could look into her eyes, if you were dumb enough to get that close, and see that no one was behind the wheel. On one memorable occasion I made it to the bathroom just ahead of her, and slammed and locked the door behind me; our prewar building was solidly built, and she pounded at the door a few times before deciding it was fruitless. The *fwoop-fwoop* of her slippers walking away; silence; a yip. The slippers came back.

"Elizabeth," she said softly through the door. I was in the bathtub, scrunched against the back wall, my head thudding hotly. "You can't be in there by yourself with the door locked. What if there was a fire?"

"There won't be a fire," I said defiantly.

Her voice turned sorrowful. "I'm sorry, Elizabeth, but I can't have you locking doors behind you. I have Mischief here, and if you don't come out, I'm going to take her down to Dr. Howell's and have her put to sleep."

My heart filled with lava; I worshipped that dog, a hyper-active Maltese with an unflattering crew cut that I maintained, with more enthusiasm than skill, with an electric beard clipper.

"He won't do it!"

Softer still. "He will, honey. I'll tell him she bit one of the kids in the building, and he'll have to. It's the law."

I knew that she was right; even other adults didn't cross my mother. Mischief whimpered. I unfolded myself from the tub and unlocked the door. She carefully put down the dog, who wisely scampered away. I didn't see her hand coming, but I did see the tile coming at me as I hit the floor.

There was always a peak to the fury, and as her anger ebbed, horror and self-flagellation flooded in to take its place. It was as if she had been possessed. As her eyes came back into focus she would dissolve into tears, keening and tugging at her hair. "I'm so sorry, Elizabeth," she'd weep. "I don't know why I do this. I don't know why I'm so vicious to you. I'm just so sorry." And I would wrap my arms around her middle, breathe in the smell of her Emeraude, and promise her that it was OK, that we were OK. The tangle in my stomach would soften and unknot, and I would relax into the sudden quiet.

We spent our summers on a working farm in the Catskills, in a tiny, hundred-occupant town called Bovina Center—I couldn't figure out at the time why the name made her laugh so hard—not far from where her stepfather, Lou, my teenage uncle Phil in tow, had circuited the hotels every summer as a Borscht Belt entertainer. To me, the farm was Narnia. I darted out of bed in the morning, snatched toast from the dining room, and was gone until sunset, unseen by adult eyes. There were goats, and rabbits, and endless litters of golden retriever puppies bred by the elderly couple who owned the farm, whom I called Oma and Opa, Grandma and Grandpa. Perfect Americana, for $300 a week.

There were hayrides, bingo, bonfires where I learned to toast marshmallows and developed a taste for scorched, liquid sugar. Mom and I joined the square dancing on the weekends, while she—strawberry-blond waves, trim figure, flirtatious eyebrows—joined the men's line in the Virginia reel, allowing me—tiny 80s shorts, scraggly hair, scabbed-up knees—to join the ladies.

Oma and Opa's morose son, Stefan, managed the buildings where guests stayed. My mother kept him supplied with the bottles of vodka he wasn't supposed to be drinking to keep us supplied with extra towels and sheets. Not that they were much to speak of. The whole place smelled slightly of damp, and the dog-and-cat-printed curtains were edged with grime.

We made friends during those summers, families visiting from cities and suburbs. They came and went for a weekend or a week, then went home to their regular lives. We stayed on for a month. No one was expecting us back at home. The families all seemed to have fathers with them, and this, I figured, *this* was the thing that made us different. Oma and Opa let every kid believe they were honorary grandparents, but they didn't invite all of them up in the winter to bunk down in their house, to follow the dogs' tracks in the snow to find the best places to sled. My mother was charming, and I was small, and it seemed the whole world wanted to adopt us.

We took the Greyhound bus, which chugged up through the mountains and left us in a dusty field, where Stefan would come pick us up in the farm truck. Like a lot of New Yorkers, my mother didn't drive, and no one we knew owned a car. The year after we acquired Mischief, we showed up at Port Authority with her carrier along with our suitcases, but dogs, it turned out, were not allowed on the buses. I sat on my suitcase and wept as the bus chugged out of the station without us, Mischief anxiously licking the tears from my face. Mom looked at me, looked at the dog, looked at the suitcases. "Come on," she said decisively. "We're going."

She strode out of the terminal with the luggage and the dog, and I followed as fast as I could. Out on Eighth Avenue, she threw up an arm. A Checker cab pulled over. She leaned in the window. "Hi, driver. What are you doing for the rest of today?" He smiled, dazzled, and she threw our suitcases into the trunk. "Get in quick before he changes his mind," she whispered out of the side of her mouth, and grinned.

He didn't change his mind. For the next few years, that same cab driver turned off his meter and drove us the four hours up the highway and over the winding roads of the mountains, then turned around and went home to the hot, shimmering city, leaving me to play in the creek and my mother to chain-smoke on the back deck reading Agatha Christie and Ngaio Marsh. At the end of the month, he'd drive up and bring us home. Dog and all.

Back at school, I fit in with my classmates best when my mother wasn't around. On each first day of school we went to Elk Candy, a hole-in-the-wall store where the elderly proprietor molded his own marzipan, to remind me that learning was sweet. "It's in the Torah!" my mother said confidently. (It's not in the Torah.) But her attitude toward school itself was sketchy at best. She thought nothing at all of yanking me out because the sun was shining, or because the snow was sticking, or because there was a good exhibit on at the Met.

When I was in first grade, we moved to a rent-stabilized three-bedroom apartment on the Upper West Side. We had nothing like enough furniture to fill it up, and I strapped on my roller skates and twirled through the empty rooms. My mother befriended the building's staff, the handymen and doormen, and as other tenants moved out or died, she'd get a discreet call on the intercom to check out the compactor room in the basement. Down we'd swoop to where the abandoned furniture and belongings had been left, waiting for trash pickup day, and we'd scavenge—a couch here, a framed landscape there, a silver cake server, a kiddush cup.

We had to keep alert, she warned. We were a minority in our own country. In kindergarten I came home full of curiosity: A boy in my class had told me he was Christian, but what did that strange word mean? To her, of course, it meant genocide. Like most Ashkenazi Jews of our time, we had lost family. Her own parents, both long dead, grew up in Queens and Brooklyn surrounded by extended families who were the only survivors—the relatives who'd stayed in the old country were murdered in the camps. Everyone who had gotten out had their back eternally to the wall and their eyes eternally open. A Christian, therefore, was someone who would report you to the gestapo as soon as look at you. Rather than say that to a five-year-old, she fished her cigarettes out of her purse and tapped one into her hand.

"Well. You know how when we go out for Chinese food, we use the lazy Susan?"

I nodded. The tabletop merry-go-round was the ultimate in fine dining, as far as I was concerned.

"And we all share food, and everyone eats off each other's plates."

"Uh-huh."

"Well," she said, satisfied, and lit up. "Christians don't do that."

Though she may have been missing some of the finer points of liturgy there, with a few decades now under my belt of reflexively offering to share my food in mixed groups and being met with either an eagerly proffered fork or a look of horror, I have to say: she wasn't wrong.

It was a secluded life in the center of a massive city. We were anonymous, a mother and daughter going about our mother-and-daughter lives. I didn't know then how many eyes were on us. A friend told me decades later, over beers, that it had taken years for her mother to leave her alone at my house; something just felt wrong about my mother, something was off, and so she dawdled behind. Playdates and parties at my house always had a big group of parents alongside, drinking coffee out of daisy-and-vine-printed cups and chatting. I thought that my mother was popular. I didn't understand that she was being monitored.

And rightly so. She was in that school building every day. She accompanied every field trip and supervised every class party, headed up every classroom team and served on every PTA. She had strong opinions about misbehavior, and about what constituted obedience. No one wanted to be within ten feet of me, since she was the chaperone who had no compunctions about screaming at her charges and terrorizing them into silence, and wherever I was, was where she was looking. When a busload of kids broke into a rousing chorus of the *Brady Bunch* theme song on the way to the Bronx Zoo, she stood up in the front, fixed her Medusa gaze on each of them in turn, and bellowed, "SHUT. UP. RIGHT. NOW." The startled driver swerved, and the song cut off as kids fell into the aisles. One time, she saw a boy on the playground being mean to me—or just thought she did—and she strode over to him, grabbed him by the throat, shoved him up against the playground wall as he choked, and hissed into his face: "*Leave my daughter alone.*"

I don't know if there was any repercussion. In retrospect, I think the grown-ups might have been scared of her too.

CHAPTER 3

The Kids Are Alright

On the Upper East Side of Manhattan, just below the 1990s-era Ninety-Sixth Street cutoff between wealth and poverty, there's a high school that looks like a prison. Or, more precisely, an armory, which is what it once was. The wall that faces Madison Avenue is slashed with arrow slits, and the squat brick building has classrooms with barely any windows at all. "They'd better have you under grow lights," my mother said, peering up at it, hands on her hips. She was bursting with pride. I was twelve years old, and I had been accepted into one of the four prestigious "specialized" high schools in New York City. It was the only one that did not focus on science and math, and the only one that started in seventh grade. It was free, but you had to first qualify to take the test, scoring in the top percentiles of the city's elementary schoolers on the citywide tests, and then beat out almost all of the competition on the Hunter test itself. Eight kids from my largely white, middle-class elementary school got in.

I chose Hunter over Chapin, a wildly expensive, tony all-girls school on the Upper East Side. I'd been awarded a full scholarship, but the luxurious building we toured—two photo labs, a fancy gym, fleets of sleek WASP-y girls streaming by in the hallways—felt like too much to me. Too much like a movie about a fish-out-of-water poor girl in a rich girls' world. I was already struggling in my Hebrew school, the only scholarship kid in a class full of the children of millionaires. I wasn't looking to add yet another place I didn't belong to the list. Mom didn't bother to hide her dismay. "Elizabeth," she said, "rich people aren't *bad*, they're just different from us. They know things, and they travel, and they've been places." She took a drag from her cigarette. "You need to *cultivate* these people."

"*Mommmm*," I moaned. "That's so hypocritical! I'm not going to be friends with people just so they can tell me about their cool trips!"

She shook her head and stubbed out her cigarette. "Suit yourself, then. You're missing out."

In my first-day-of-school picture, standing awkwardly against my white pressboard desk, I'm wearing a long denim skirt, white Keds, and a white blouse printed with fruit and tied at the waist. I look apprehensive, anxious. The photo is prescient. I tried to kill myself that spring.

Middle school and I did not get along. My classmates thought I was a weirdo, and they were right. They wanted to know what was wrong with me, and I couldn't have told them for all the money in the world.

But there was plenty. I was garden-variety middle-school ugly, with a soft, ill-formed face, giant silver braces, and frizzy hair. Not actually any better or worse than anyone around me, but every teenager feels like there's something inherently, personally, Wrong with them, and I kept getting confirmation. A dead father—Surely I meant grandfather? No?—and kids scattering like spiders in front of my mother when she strode into the school. There legitimately *was* something wrong in my house, but I didn't have a name for it. All the Scholastic book fair books about abuse showed kids with their arms in slings and hair arranged over bruises; she rarely hit me, though, man, did she wallop when she did. I told people the truth, but it came out halfhearted and whiny. "She's really strict." "She yells a lot." I didn't say: I'm afraid of her. I didn't say: when she gets angry, something Terminator-red shines behind her eyes.

I ran around with a set of equally quiet, slightly weird girls. Two of my close friends were recent Taiwanese immigrants, studious, with sly senses of humor; on weekends we went to the ritzy toy store FAO Schwarz and shuffled through the Sanrio racks, cooing over sticker sets and sweet-smelling pens. I was age-inappropriately obsessed with a blank-faced duck called Pekkle. Our fourth was a white girl from the Bronx, whose divorced parents were an acupuncturist and an acupressurist, mysterious professions I couldn't keep straight, though there seemed to be a lot of statues of Buddha involved. She wore dream-catcher earrings and tie-dyed shirts, and I sneakily tried to emulate everything about her, hoping that I could fake being normal if I just Joanna-fied everything I did.

On the half-Wednesdays each month when teachers had their conferences, we walked ten blocks down to Eighty-Sixth Street and Lexington, an intersection that had everything we needed: a McDonald's, an HMV, and a Barnes & Noble. We couldn't afford anything there, of course, but that strip of Lexington had a street-carnival atmosphere. Enterprising entrepreneurs jockeyed for space with the three-card monte players, setting up folding tables piled with dollar books, or incense, or gloves. I didn't realize until my own publishing days that the books were stolen out of the Barnes & Noble dumpsters out back. Bookstores operate more or less on consignment and can return any inventory they don't sell. They only have to ship back the covers for mass market paperbacks to get credit, since paper costs more to send than it's worth to resell, and the street sellers handily rescued the half-naked books and sold them ten feet from the store's front door. I went through piles of science fiction and fantasy and dramatic true crime and it-happened-to-me adventure tales.

Despite having a few friends, I was a social failure. Mom knew something was going wonkus, but couldn't figure out what it was. She had been popular, after all. Why was I so unhappy? What was wrong with me? And how could she architect a solution?

Appropriately for a lawyer, "retired" or otherwise: with threats.

Dear [School Principal],
    Over a month ago, my daughter Elizabeth was assaulted by [Hapless Adolescent], another Hunter 7th grader, in the hall at Hunter. Elizabeth was standing at her locker, showing her collection of "New Kids on the Block" memorabilia to a girlfriend when Hapless passed with a group of his friends. Calling Elizabeth names, he grabbed a handful of her posters and ran down the hall with them. Elizabeth pursued him to recover her property; the boy tore up what he had taken. Remembering that she had left her locker door open, Elizabeth returned to find the remnants of her collection destroyed.

I went to the school on the following Monday morning
and reported the incident to [Overworked Teacher], who
immediately took me to [Vice Principal]'s office. I told VP
in the strongest terms that I expected appropriate action
to be taken, including a letter of apology from Hapless to
Elizabeth, notification of Hapless's parents, and restoration
of all the items stolen and destroyed.

VP wanted to get Hapless's side of the story, which I
agreed was absolutely fair. She assured me that the matter would be appropriately and promptly dealt with by the
school authorities. Because of these assurances, I did not
report the incident to the police. [Ed. note: Yes. The police.
I know. But wait! It gets better.]

Now, a month later, nothing whatever has been done.
When I spoke to VP yesterday, she laughed and said she'd
sent a notice to Hapless's homeroom class, instructing him
to come to her office, but that he had not responded. She
further stated that there is a "policy" against removing a
child from class.

This is a lame excuse and a cavalier approach to a very
serious incident. Like all other 7th graders, Hapless has 10
free periods, 5 lunch periods, and 5 homeroom periods—20
non-class opportunities every week for 4 weeks in which VP
might have required his presence. Furthermore, his behavior is sufficiently alarming to justify his losing class time to
deal with it.

The fact is that VP has treated the entire episode as
a sort of "boys will be boys" joke. As I left her office last
month, she called out to me that I should be glad I don't
have a boy. What exactly does this mean? That the boys
at Hunter (and elsewhere) have some sort of license to

assault and vandalize, and it's just their good old testosterone that's to blame?

To make matters worse, Elizabeth has told me that Overworked Teacher later joked that perhaps Hapless did this because "he has a crush on you." What an appalling commentary on sexism at Hunter! I thought it was no longer acceptable to tell women that abuse is one of the ways in which men may legitimately express their "affection." I do not want my daughter being misled by authority figures at Hunter into the acceptance of aggression as "love." Aggression is a violent assault, and it cannot be justified.

I assume Elizabeth did not report this incident immediately because her previous experience with being rather brutally "hazed" by a large group of upperclassmen during her first weeks at Hunter had given her the very clear impression that this conduct is tolerated within the school. In any event, I do not want anyone at Hunter discussing this with her except in my presence, since she is learning some "lessons" there which are totally unacceptable in her value system. And what kind of message is Hapless receiving when his behavior has no consequences and he can even ignore a summons from VP?

I expect that you will now immediately investigate and take appropriate action within the next two days. Please let me know exactly what is being done. Should there be a further failure to resolve this situation, I shall be forced to pursue other remedies.

Kindly acknowledge receipt of this letter by signing the enclosed copy and returning it to me.

Signed, J. S. Scheier, JD

There's so much to unpack here. The cold legal language, which raises the hackles on my neck thirty years later, and I'm not even the addressee. The wild, incredible overreaction to a few pop posters shredded and a nasty comment from a twelve-year-old. The threats. The privilege of viewing an incident in which no one ever touched me as a violent assault. Knowing what I now know about her life, of course, I think I know what she was thinking. She was *not* going to let what had happened to her happen to me, even if it meant calling a barely adolescent boy, in the most high-minded of terms, a little shit.

And yet.

I can't disagree with the sentiment. The kid was just dumb, but those adults definitely pulled a "boys will be boys" on the wrong woman. If someone did this to my daughter, I wouldn't send this letter, but I would write it over and over in my head, furiously, before falling asleep. I'm horrified but also, reluctantly, kind of proud. She didn't know how to sheathe her claws, but sometimes she used them to good effect.

This was classic Judith Scheier: the right idea, but an execution that veered wildly off the rails.

The fallout was, predictably, worse than the initial crime. The story of the tangle slalomed around the hallways, and I went from being invisible to being Something Wrong; not only a snitch, but one with a crazy mother, and who knew? Maybe crazy myself. So I put my head way down and kept my mouth shut about everything else that happened that year. My classmates scented blood and went after it. On one occasion, I intercepted a cartoon that was circulating in my social studies class, featuring me being raped by a German shepherd; according to the caption, it was one of a series.

By the end of the year, I'd had it. I was done. My secret was out: I was irretrievably broken. Entirely unfixable. Now everyone knew it. Nothing left for it but suicide. I got down to business.

I chose pills. There are a surprising number of pills in your average medicine cabinet. Painkillers, a couple of different brands. Allergy medication. Decongestants. That last dose of antibiotics you forgot to take for that UTI that one time. They add up to a lot. I took all of them.

That turned out to be my mistake. You take forty, your system overwhelms and you die; you take four hundred, your stomach revolts and you throw most of them up. Which I did. For hours. Crouched on the bathroom floor on a fluffy yellow bathmat. Between heaves, I dutifully read my English homework, which was—I still remember—John Steinbeck's novella *The Pearl*. Why? Who knows. Maybe some part of me never believed I would die, and feared being in trouble if I went back to class without my homework.

I woke up hours later, back in my bed, the scratching sound of a long claw etching the wall next to me, the bump of a carapace the size of a Rottweiler shifting under the mattress. The sheer white curtains rustled in the soft, damp air coming in the window. In the wan light of the streetlamps, I saw the air shift and the walls ripple. There was something beneath them, something bubbling up the plaster and paint without breaking through. I whimpered and gathered my nightgown under me, inched my heels under my body, and made a jump for the middle of the floor, out of reach of the straining walls. The air rushed in as the plaster split and I ran, heart in my throat, for the door and my mother's bedroom. She opened the covers for me and turned over with a grunt.

The walls stayed still for a blessed moment and then swelled. A man's silhouette leaned in through the connected bathroom's window, hung, and dropped to the floor. More climbed in from the ceiling and the walls. I knew there was no way I would leave that room alive, and I gathered up my meager courage and started singing, tremulously, the Shema, the central prayer of Judaism—*Hear O Israel, the Lord is our God, the Lord is One.* The last words that are supposed to cross your lips before death. "Elizabeth! Cool it with the Shema," my mother said sharply, wrenched from sleep.

A chill came over me. "Are you with them?" I asked.

"What? *What?* With whom?"

Christ. She *was* with them. My own mother had opened our home to assassins who were trying to kill me.

I jumped from the bed and ran down the hall and wrenched open the lock and the deadbolt. I raced barefoot down the hallway and down five flights of stairs and through the lobby, past the startled doorman and halfway down the block, night-gown wafting behind me, before passersby caught me and brought me home.

I woke up in the morning to shifting walls and lazily spinning colors. No longer afraid—I had accepted that I was going to die, probably painfully, and probably at the hands of her mysterious, window-climbing friends—I installed myself on the couch in the dining room and spoke to the ceiling. Spidery legs surfaced through the paint, and the ceiling light fixture lowered and raised. My mother's best friend, a doctor, came over, took one look at me, and called an ambulance.

I remember, blearily, sitting in a plastic bucket seat in the hospital with a cup full of activated charcoal, my mother frantically trying to get me to drink it. I remember my ankles and wrists being restrained to a hospital bed, and screaming that if they hurt me, my cop boyfriend would get revenge. (I didn't have a boyfriend, obviously, and I didn't know any cops.) I woke up in the middle of the night in a dark, quiet room, attached to an IV, still tied down, while a nurse silently observed me from a chair in the corner, her eyes flinty and accusatory. I remember a doctor coming in the next morning and saying jovially, "Wow, you sure were feisty when you came in!" I didn't know what "feisty" meant—did he mean something sexual? What had I *done?*—and I cringed in humiliation.

They kept me for seventy-two hours' observation and released me into my mother's promise of therapy and monitoring. I followed her silently down the hall, scuffing my sneakers so they squeaked. We stopped in billing, and I slumped in a chair while she talked to a woman sitting at a desk behind a half-door. "Insurance?" the woman said briskly. "Self-pay," my mother said. There was a pause. The woman leaned out of the half-door and said, hesitantly, "She was here for a while. There was an ambulance ride. It's going to be expensive."

"Self-pay," my mother repeated, her voice strained but firm.

I don't know if we had any insurance. She certainly didn't have a job. But what I know now is that my mother had signed me into the hospital under a fake Social Security number, determined that this episode wouldn't follow me through the rest of my life. As an adult, I looked back on that day and thought that I must be misremembering: surely faking a Social was too much, even for her. But no. On maternity leave with my second child, I sorted through old boxes and found school records with my fake Social Security number on them. "Well *fuck,*" I said to sleeping one-month-old David, sprawled froggy-style on his playmat. "She pulled it off."

She pulled off a truly extraordinary number of things, especially for a woman whose mood was unreliable at best and who had only the most tenuous idea of how other people functioned in the world. She lived in a luxury neighborhood in one of the most expensive cities on earth for decades without working a single day. She won over an astonishing array of people—the maintenance staff at my elementary school, the office staff at the chichi synagogue who slipped her free High Holy Days tickets, the doorman who visited her daily for decades and sent her flowers on her birthday. The fact that she fooled so many people should have made me feel better that she fooled me too. It doesn't.

When I came home from the hospital, my bedroom door had been taken off its hinges, and it stayed that way for the next year. The bathroom door—the scene of the crime—was still there, so I don't know what she thought she was accomplishing. I went to a few desultory sessions with a hospital-ordered therapist, who decided that I was more fearful of another hallucinatory episode than I was of living, and released me. I went back to school, more sullen than before, and ignored the looks and muttering as best I could.

But there was a new glint in my eye. For the first time, my mother was not the one with all the cards. I had something she needed: my own life. I could hold myself hostage. She backed off her rage, locking *herself* in the bathroom for a change when she couldn't control it, beating the walls. One night, she came into my room to yell when I was typing spitefully away on the computer. I stood up quickly from my chair. She fell back, suddenly speechless. We both saw what neither of us had realized until that moment: I had grown taller than she was.

It was two years before she hit me again. After one of our

knock-down drag-outs, I slammed out of the apartment, pausing to knock a snarling wooden Japanese mask from the wall next to the door. It hit the floor and cracked, and I fled, panicked. I got on the 7 train and made it all the way out to Flushing, to the home of a friend, a girl whose own mother beat her around the shoulders with a hanger when her grades weren't good enough. She would understand.

They let me in and Erica and I huddled in their shared bedroom, heads together, as her mother hesitated, debating what to do with me; finally, she called my mother to tell her I was alive and well. Mom must have almost fallen over her feet getting in a cab, and an hour later the four of us convened in a nearby Chinese restaurant to discuss what was to be done with me. I refused to go home. My friend's mother pleaded in stilted English. My friend held my hand tight under the table, cautioning: don't startle them.

"This is enough, Elizabeth," Mom said tightly. "You've inconvenienced everyone with your little temper tantrum. It's time to go home now. Come on."

I stared at the tablecloth. "No."

Mom slammed the table and heaved to her feet. I jumped up; she stepped toward me and I ran, again, dodging curious waiters and passersby, her voice behind me: *you get back here*. Cars flashed by, and the elevated 7 train rumbled overhead, faces obscured behind the fogged-up windows.

I walked for hours. I got as far as the highway before a squad car blooped its siren and pulled up next to me. I don't know where I thought I was going, but "somewhere else" sounded pretty fucking great. For the first time, I thought: *There are other places. I could be in one of them.*

The police brought me home. They marched me from the

squad car into the building, the doorman and the handyman exchanging a significant look. "You can't *leave* me there," I said to the officers in the elevator, my voice hitching and hiccupping. "She'll kill me." "Naaaaaaah," said the officer, comfortably. "These are hard years, kid. I get it. We've all been there. But she's your mother and she loves you. It'll be OK." I imagine his sympathy was limited; a well-fed white kid running away from a newly gentrified neighborhood and a prewar building. Teenagers and parents have fights all the time, right?

Officer Nonchalance rang the bell and stepped back. The slippers approached. The door opened, and I saw only a quick glimpse of her cold face before she reached out, grabbed me by the hair, and smacked my head into the doorframe. I fell to the floor and laced my fingers over my neck, knees tight to my chest. No one moved for a long moment. I heard the officers' weight shift. They muttered uncomfortably and confirmed her identity and mine, and my head still locked to my knees, I heard them get back on the elevator—it hadn't even had time to return to the lobby.

The door closed between me and the world. A good lesson, learned young: The cavalry isn't coming. There is no one to save you but you. I kept myself locked in a closet until her rage subsided. That time.

❖ ❖ ❖

I fell in love for the first time when I was fifteen. He was a guitar player (aren't they all) with dirty blond curls and flinty, cold-blue eyes. He wrote poetry and song lyrics for a band called Lack Thereof (as in "talent or," get it, haw haw), and pitched for our high school's baseball team. I thought he was the most magical guy who had ever lived, largely because he liked me when I was pretty sure that "sack of shit" would be a generous self-description. His name was Brian, but he went— and when I recount this now I want to shake my younger self, hard—by Billy, after Billy Joel. (Yes. I *know*.)

Here's the thing about city adolescence: the places to fool around in are much rarer than in the suburbs. We don't have cars, so no backseats. We don't have basements, so no musty cast-off couches. No woods, no riverbanks. We made out furiously in Central Park, but public parks are intentionally designed without potentially dangerous secluded spots, so more often than not we were driven off by righteous parents of toddlers or catcalling older men. On a bright fall afternoon in October, on a day I knew my mother would be auditing a class, I skipped my afternoon classes and snuck him home with me, past the eyebrow-raised doorman and into my empty apartment. I skipped the tour—who had time?—and we got right to it in my bed. I was sitting astride him wearing only my jeans when we heard a key in the front door. My whole chest clenched painfully.

Faintly, I thought I heard voices from the front hall.

I leapt off him and he ran, naked, into my bathroom. I pitched his clothes after him and slammed the door. A heavy tread in the hallway, and my mother appeared. I had a bra on and was struggling into a new T-shirt.

"What are you doing home?"

I swallowed. My hands were shaking, visibly.

"My lab was canceled."

Her eyes narrowed. "Why are you changing shirts?"

"I spilled soda on mine."

She strode past me and wrenched my closet door open. Then the other. She pushed past me and got the bathroom door open just as Billy got his shirt over his head. She grabbed him by the shoulder and marched him silently out of the bedroom, down the hall, and out the front door. The sound of the slam was so loud that I wondered, briefly, if the door had broken.

She appeared back in the doorway. I could smell the rage building in her. Crazy-rage smells crackling and mineral, like airplane bathrooms, like cocaine. I tried to back up against the wall, but she grabbed my arm and threw me to the floor.

"You *whore*. You filthy *whore*. In my house! In my *house*."

I crab-scuttled back. Her eyes jittered frantically around the room and landed on the bulletin board above my bed. She crossed the room in two leaps and started pulling photos of my friends down, ripping them in half.

"You won't need these anymore where you're going. You won't need memories of your life. Your life is *over*."

She threw the scraps to the bed and ran out of the room. I followed. Not seeing her was worse; when she was in the room, at least I had my eye on her. She was just as capable of reappearing with a gun as with a spatula or a vase or the dog, neck freshly broken. She turned on her heel, grabbed me by the elbow, and spun me against the wall, where my shoulder hit with a thud. She slammed through the apartment, yanking all the phone extensions out of the jacks except for the one in her room. There would be no calling for help.

Throughout that long night, she periodically threw my door wide and hissed invectives at me. On one trip she threw a duffel bag in the door and demanded I start packing, right then. She was going to send me to Arizona to my aunt and uncle, where I'd never see my friends—or *that boy*—again.

When she finally fell asleep, I boxed up letters from Billy, my diaries, and some other odds and ends I couldn't live without. I crept down to the lobby, heart clanging in my throat, and asked the night doorman to hold them until a friend could come pick them up. He looked at me with sympathy and tucked the box carefully under his arm.

I didn't go to Arizona. The next day, my godmother Shannon picked me up and took me to her home in New Jersey, where I took up residence in the guest room. Every morning, she drove me down to the ferry terminal at six a.m., and we sang along with the British *Les Mis* soundtrack at the top of our lungs, tunelessly and joyfully. My shoulders settled in a new low spot under my neck where, I realized, they'd belonged the whole time.

I took the commuter ferry across the Hudson to school, the prow of the ship breaking the ice as the winter turned cold. My mother and the guidance counselor worked out a system where I was required to sign in to each class so that she could be sure I wasn't cutting. My teachers looked me up and down sorrowfully, half the time forgetting to have anywhere for me to sign in at all. My most strict and imposing teacher stopped me in the hallway, and said slowly and meaningfully, "We're supposed to report in on you. I hope you know we don't have anything to report, and won't, no matter what happens." I stared at the floor and thanked her in a small voice. Someone had seen me. Someone had *seen*.

For the first time, I understood that my mother, too, was being seen. And that someone knew that something was wrong. The teachers weren't complying with this over-the-top surveillance plan because they agreed that I was a troublemaker who needed watching. No. They were complying to keep her calm. To some extent, to keep me safe. It was an electric realization. Everything was crashing down around my head, but finally, someone *knew*. Someone was watching.

In her mind, she sent me away to save me from her own rage. I sometimes recognize this double-personality game in myself, the better self playing defense for the worse. Some part of her knew that if I stayed there she would hurt me too badly. That she might kill me. But I was a teenager, so I focused on the immediate drama of it. I had been *kicked out of the house*. I was not supposed to have phone access, or get mail, or have any social time—my godmother got special permission for me to go to my camp reunion, fierce on the phone. "*Judith*, this is the most important event for her this year, it's like the *prom*; don't stick to this so tightly, you'll always regret it." But Shannon and Joe took a spirit-of-the-law approach and treated me like a beloved visiting cousin, not a pariah.

The thought of next summer's camp session was what kept me going. Buck's Rock sits just north of New York City in rural Connecticut, a haven for artsy kids where dubious social skills are no barrier to making friends. Some were close enough to see in the city; my friend Arie was at Hunter too, the year below me, though he was cool and I was the loserest of losers. He spent his summer days camping it up in the clown shop; I scribbled in an Adirondack chair in the publications shop, writing blisteringly humiliating poetry and impassioned essays on subjects that merited no passion at all. I wore overalls and bandanas and boots, because it was the 90s, and felt like the most unfortunate, unattractive soul in human history. We talked in the hallways while I was in New Jersey Exile, shoulders against the lockers, and my teachers passed by and averted their eyes; there would be no reporting my interaction with a certified male human being.

Three months after she kicked me out, Mom had had enough therapy. Or enough Entenmann's coffee cake. Or had screamed herself out. I have no idea. I was allowed to come home, and my life resumed largely without mention of what had happened, although I was grounded for life. She was considering hiring a Barnard student to follow me in the streets, she said, and I would *never*—her eyebrows raised significantly—know when it would happen.

I was no longer allowed to close my bedroom door.

One of the first strands in the rope that bound her to me stretched tight, whined, and broke. A shuttered window had been broken open, and there were eyes on us now. She had gone to my principal and my teachers with a shopping list of my sins and what she considered a rational plan for resolving them, but for the first time, I knew that outside parties were seeing what I saw: a frantic, manic outlier whose anger was far out of sync with circumstance. The something wrong in my house wasn't *me*, a revelation that thrilled and frightened me. My friends who hadn't met her suddenly saw that I hadn't been making it up all along; she was not just a strict single parent, but something different. Something to be cautious of.

I muscled through the rest of high school with my elbows out, angry and defensive. If I'd been rebellious before, I tripled my efforts now. I felt not a shred of guilt about it. If most aspects of a normal social life were forbidden, why trust her judgment at all? I was going to get away with every damn thing I could get away with. I cut classes to be with my boyfriend, I lied about where I was, and I stayed up late in AOL chat rooms talking to god-knows-who about god-knows-what. It was freeing. One day, one day soon, I'd be out, and I planned to flee for college as if shot out of a cannon, a rousing John Philip Sousa march as the soundtrack.

When college acceptance letters rolled in, the most financial aid came from a small women's college outside Philadelphia. I wasn't crazy about the idea; I'd wanted to go to a giant
state school somewhere, a university where I could fade into the
background and disappear. But we had no money, and even Bryn
Mawr's generous package required an annual letter-writing
campaign explaining, patiently, that the zero on the "expected
family contribution" line on the FAFSA form meant exactly
what it said. There was no money waiting to be scraped out
from behind the couch cushions, and I was a book geek hoping
to go into publishing, a field that would barely cover a decent
stash of ramen, let alone the levels of loan they were suggesting.
Eventually, they always relented.

It's bonkers, isn't it? We had no money at all, weren't even
working class, in the sense that no one in my home worked.
But we benefited from the patina of nonexistent wealth. When
she could keep her cool, my mother sounded like what she
was—a highly educated white woman who expected to be listened to. And she knew how to play the game. She understood
the college admissions process. She marched my sullen ass
through the applications, and she harassed the financial aid
people until they gave me more money just to make her go
away. The dollar value of her ability to play a person much
fancier than she actually was turned out to be the price of four
years at an expensive school. I worked thirty hours a week in
the dining hall, determined to put something away beyond the
tuition bills.

On school breaks I worked at the flagship Bloomingdale's
on Fifty-Ninth Street. In winter I served the Christmas crowds,
folding and refolding cashmere sweaters and memorizing the

same thirteen Christmas songs that played on a loop. (I still feel a surge of claustrophobic, merino-scented rage every time I hear the opening chimes of "All I Want for Christmas Is You," the most loathsome song ever written, I will brook no argument on this.) In the summer—prom, graduation, and wedding season—I worked in the formal dress section. I fitted bored or anxious teen girls into their prom dresses, found the rare off-the-rack size 14s for drag queens, and handed dozens of women tissues as they burst into tears over dress sizes that no longer fit and undeserving sisters who were getting married first. I learned one of the most body image–enhancing lessons of my life standing behind a thousand women eyeing themselves distrustfully in the mirror: mirrors are misrepresenting assholes and you always, *always* look better in person than you do in your reflection.

We made six percent commission on everything customers bought, and got it docked right back for everything they returned. Sometimes you spent two hours with a customer who ended up buying nothing; once, a bride walked in with the style number of a dress she'd seen in a magazine and ordered it sight unseen for every one of her fourteen bridesmaids. We got cash kickbacks—a few dollars, but everything counted when returns could wipe out your entire paycheck— for opening store credit cards, and I sold that shit *hard*. If you met me during the years 1996–1998, I signed you up for a Bloomingdale's card.

That money bought me the few thousand in tuition I owed after grants and loans. It also covered most of the basics: never quite enough shampoo and toothpaste, and food over breaks, which I spent living at my boyfriend Torsten's, a kind-hearted editor I met during a paid summer internship at a science fiction magazine. After my mother's revelation on the couch—my suspicions of her lies revealed, and the truth worse than I'd known—we'd circled each other warily, the newly out story between us. She had fooled me so completely that I no longer took anything she said on its face. The apartment rang with mistrust. It was a relief to have somewhere else to go.

CHAPTER 4

That's How the Light Gets In

"I was married when you were born, but not to your father," she said, and the room was quiet for a long moment.

"OK," I said finally. "So . . . was Kurt my father?" She'd divorced her first husband after ten years of marriage, and I'd met him once, when I was four or five; he gave me a small cork-stoppered jar full of colored shells, which I treasured. I couldn't remember what he looked like, or if there was any resemblance.

"No, for goodness' sake. Don't be ridiculous." She caught herself. "I'm sorry. This is just hard to say."

I waited.

"Kurt and I divorced when I was only in my thirties. I know that sounds ancient to you, but I was still a young woman. I wanted to be with someone, you know? Loneliness is terrible." She coughed, hard; her four-pack-a-day habit had crept to six while I was away.

"When I met Merrill, I was just charmed by him. We fell in love right away and he wanted to get married immediately. I thought it was romantic. Elizabeth, don't be stupid like me. Don't ever just take someone at their word."

The irony gods inexplicably failed to strike her down on the spot. "We got married in front of a judge, and on the drive home from the ceremony, he pulled over to the side of the road and popped the hood. He said there were voices calling out to him from inside the engine, and he had to stop them." I boggled at her. "He started hitting me that week. I couldn't believe what was happening and I didn't know what to do or who to call. My mother was dead and Lou was gone with Phil. I finally called the police when he tried to strangle me with the phone cord in the kitchen."

She called the police from that same innocent beige wall model from which I made all my childhood phone calls. But it was the early 70s, and the new term "domestic violence" was still considered to be a private matter between a man and his wife. The police took her statement, warned him not to let his temper get the better of him, and left.

She finally locked him out, installing double bolts on the door of that Yorkville apartment where I was born. He pursued her for a while, and she refused him. He died, never having spoken to her again or filed for divorce, when I was sixteen.

Which means, for those of you playing along at home, that until I was a junior in high school, my mother was still married—to a man whose name I'd never heard.

Not too long after Merrill left, she was sunbathing in Central Park when a blond head appeared above her, features shadowed out by the sun. He looked to her like one of the bronzed Greek gods in illustrated books of mythology. He asked for part of her *New York Times*. Flattered—at thirty-eight, she was ten years older than he was—she gave it to him.

They began a romance, just as whirlwind as the one in the lie she'd originally told—they were together "maybe six months or a year," she said—based on their mutual loneliness and depression. They listened to Simon & Garfunkel's *Sounds of Silence* together over and over, gloomily. I started to understand how and why she had kept him secret from her friends; this did not sound like the kind of couple that got invited to a lot of parties.

At some stage in the relationship, when she hadn't heard from him in a week, she finally called his apartment. His wife, from whom he was separated—now his widow, rather than his almost-ex—picked up the phone. He had jumped from the rooftop of his building. She was cleaning up after the funeral. He had never mentioned my mother to his family, and they didn't know to inform her. The newspaper article announcing his suicide never mentioned his name.

His name, by the way, was indeed Warren. Not Warren Steven Livingston, he of the nice Jewish name and the unlucky timing at a red light. But Warren Frank Luther, married man, suicide.

She'd known he was troubled, but not how much. She hung up the phone in silence, alone once more, and retreated to her room. Months later, her doddering but trusted doctor diagnosed her with a tumor on her pituitary gland. A dedicated hypochondriac, she'd been waiting for news like this her whole life, and, gravely, she got on a plane to California on a farewell tour to visit my uncle, his wife, and their little boys. My Aunt Kathy, not a particularly worldly woman but considerably smarter than my mother in some very important ways, took one look at my mother, and said, "Honey, you're not dying. You are *pregnant*."

This was—again—the 70s. She'd spent years on the kind of pill with no week off in the middle for your period; she was on a hefty dose of progesterone the whole month long. She had just gone off it when she met Warren and was using a diaphragm, so it never occurred to her to be concerned that her period was still AWOL.

(Public service announcement: *do not rely on a diaphragm*.)

She returned to New York, stricken. I was an adult when I finally asked why she didn't abort me when she found out she was pregnant. She had never been a big fan of kids, my father was dead, she was more or less alone and getting more so every year. *Roe v. Wade* was just a few years old, and much less besieged than it is today. She was independent and had savings from her decade working as a lawyer. She could have flown anywhere in the world that would have performed the procedure. "Well," she said slowly, "by the time I realized I was pregnant, I was almost five months along. I started feeling you kicking when I was still in shock."

After two of my own pregnancies, I get this. The stomach-flu stage is one thing, but the tap of the world's tiniest pencil eraser against your abdomen is unmistakable and unforgettable. I can see how it made a hard decision infinitely harder.

And so she didn't abort me. She planned to adopt me out. As a newborn I was agreeably quiet, clutched close to her "even when I went to the bathroom!" At twelve days, convinced I was mute, she poked me with a diaper pin to make sure. I was not mute, as the neighbors can attest.

And so she kept me. She never regretted this decision. There were many days (and many years) when I did.

She finished the story and fell silent. I was sitting cross-legged on the couch, my book forgotten on the floor. In a chair by the living room door, she studied her hands clasped in the lap of her purple crepe housedress.

I had no idea what to say. I had a million half-formed questions, none of them ready to make it out of my mouth in any kind of coherent way. My head was a gridlock of emotions: pity for her, sadness for Warren, surprise that my cattle prod of a mother had been beaten by a man she was married to. But mostly I was just plain shocked. A whole other husband. A whole other person in my mother's life. If she had been hit by a truck while he was still alive, would some in-case-of-emergency notification have popped up, and some mystery man have appeared? How had she left out this salient piece of information? How did I never know?

And of course, the eternal consideration when dealing with Judith Scheier: Was a single word of this even true?

"I." I cleared my throat. "I'm sorry. That all sounds . . . that sounds hard."

She nodded, examining her fingernails.

"Why did you tell me he died in a car accident, though? Is that . . . better? I don't understand."

She shook her head. "I didn't know how to talk about suicide to a little kid. That's not an easy thing to explain. And then when you were older, you were depressed, and I didn't want to give you any ideas." She shot me a pained look, and I thought guiltily of the choked sobbing I'd heard from her room in the nights after I came back from the hospital, rolled into a tight, sleepless ball in my yellow-sheeted twin bed. "And I didn't want you to know where he died. I was afraid you'd make a shrine out of it."

(In fairness, she was probably right about that.)

"But why did you make up a name? Why didn't you just tell me his real name?"

The first glimmer of impatience crossed her face. "Honey, you have to understand, this was a different time. Single mothers lost custody of their kids. All. The. Time. There was a big story going on in the news just when I found out I was pregnant, about a pair of wealthy grandparents taking a baby away from a single mother, and that wasn't going to happen to me. I was going to fight to keep you no matter what!" Her eyes flared. Somewhere in there, she was fending off a ravaging horde of custody officers and kleptocratic grandparents with a dagger, shielding me behind her. "I couldn't risk you trying to find him. I couldn't risk you trying to find his *family*. You don't know what kind of people these are."

"You're right," I said as evenly as I could manage. "I don't."

On a roll, she missed my tone. "Anyway, it didn't matter. He was dead and I couldn't bring him back. I wanted to give you a father, but he was gone." Her mouth crumpled. She had lost something, too. Not a love—it was clear that she barely remembered this blond paramour who picked her up in Central Park—but another adult, a person who could have been *around*. Who could have helped her make decisions, and listened to her, and provided some balance and some ballast. I thought, with shame that it had not occurred to me before, how lonely it must have been to raise me by herself. Lonely and hard. I had not been peaches to live with a lot of those years, either. But she had stuck it out, and she had indeed fought to keep me. Whether for her sake or mine, I couldn't say.

I opened my mouth to ask more questions, but she stood up briskly. "Well. I just wanted you to know. So now you know."

The fuck I did.

But now I *wanted* to.

Now he was within reach. His story was beginning to fill out—a hair color, the fact that he had enough game to pick up a sunbathing woman engrossed in a newspaper. He'd had parents of his own, my *grandparents*, a concept I had never considered over the more immediate absence. We had both tried to put a permanent end to our own sadness, but my recalcitrant stomach had given me a grace the concrete sidewalk hadn't given him. I wanted to weep and rage and throw up, all at once. I sat awake and alone in my bedroom all night, my head blazing with betrayal.

I had always suspected. Her stories were clearly bullshit. But now I knew for sure. Now she had *told* me she'd been lying. And I had just enough information to know what I didn't know, and all I could do was hope it was real. The man who wasn't there was materializing over the horizon, no longer just a fuzzy blond outline, but blood, bone, and trauma. He had been a real person, and he'd had no idea he'd conceived me.

If he had, would he still have jumped?

I shut down that line of thinking. That way lay madness.

But for the first time, I started thinking seriously about looking for him.

✦ ✦ ✦

She still called me multiple times a day, the blinking red message light a permanent fixture on my dorm answering machine. I started to ignore most of the calls. I felt no responsibility to her, not yet; I was supporting myself, after all, and she was still capable of taking care of herself day to day. Slowly, I started to see what the world might look like through only my own eyes, without her caustic voice in my head. I worked long hours in the dining center and studied late in the library and tried to imagine a future with only myself as a priority. It was a misty vision, but a thrilling one.

The next summer, I was preparing to leave for my junior year abroad in London, paid for grudgingly by my close-to-full scholarship. Furious after a fight, Mom had threatened to put my beloved Mischief to sleep if I didn't find her another home while I was gone. "Why should I take care of *your* dog while *you* go gallivanting across the globe?" she yelled. I pounded the pavement looking for somewhere for her to live for that year. Tor was willing to take her, but when I brought her over for a trial run, she yapped incessantly while he was at work, unaccustomedly lonely. His building didn't allow pets. Desperate, I called the vet; would he remove her vocal cords? As an absolute last resort, he would. The tone of his voice made clear that he thought I was probably an animal abuser and certainly out of my damn mind.

Who else did I know who was a grown-up?

Aha: Jim.

Jim lived in a walk-up near Lincoln Center, a tiny, must-and-leather-smelling apartment crammed floor to ceiling with piles of books. To get to his bedroom-slash-office, you edged your way past a series of bookshelves and hugged the wall to turn the corner. I adored the white ceramic elephants, trunks raised, that flanked the radiator. A drafting desk filled most of the tiny bedroom, and I had spent hours perched on his ample lap, rapt, watching his pencil feather out a mermaid's hair, slice out the lines of a Roman soldier's helmet.

When I was very young I'd been convinced he actually was my father. My mother clearly adored him, and he was gruffly affectionate to me, avuncular, ready to spend hours drawing according to my most exacting and demanding specifications. He hand-lettered my birthday party invitations in writing that looked like bubbly copperplate. His cards to me are all signed "Lovable Jim."

He was, indeed, lovable. He was also a short, dark-complexioned brunet with a reddish beard, so I'd always known it was a long shot. When my mother slammed down the phone one night and announced we were no longer speaking to Jim— "He's passive-aggressive!" she said furiously, a wholly unfamiliar but threatening-sounding phrase—I wasn't surprised. I mostly gave up on the fantasy of the secret father, nearby but hidden.

I hadn't seen him in ten years by the time I rang his bell; he sounded the same, his voice sonorous and deep. When he heard my name, he was clearly taken aback, but invited me up. I went up the stairs with Mischief panting obligingly in my arms, my heart thudding.

The apartment still looked the same, still smelled like pipe smoke. This is the magic of rent-stabilized buildings in New York: condo buildings may shoot up alongside, lobbies may transform into shiny, foreign-autocrat-beckoning rent traps, the CTown down the street may become a Whole Foods, but up a few flights are the same middle-class stalwarts who've been there since the 1960s and who've been paying tiny rent increases ever since. They don't renovate or redecorate; why would you put money into something you don't own? They don't buy a ton of new stuff; where would it go? All these time capsules of old-school artists still exist, somewhere at the tops of sixth-floor walk-ups, their tenants Collyer-brothered in between dusty-smelling bookcases.

Jim hugged me carefully, invited me in, asked me to sit

down, suggested with embarrassment that I not go into the bathroom. I took a careful seat on the leather couch, propped on the edge with the dog carrier slung around my neck, Mischief looking patiently around. I made small talk—way too little small talk for even a modicum of courtesy—and asked if he'd take the dog. He regretfully refused; he had increasing trouble getting up and down the stairs, he said, and didn't think he could walk her. *She's used to a litter box*, I almost said, but caught myself in time. Looking back, I can't believe my own chutzpah—asking someone I hadn't seen in a decade to dog-sit for a year while I went adventuring on the college's dime overseas. My only defense is that I was twenty. And kind of an asshole.

We looked at each other and smiled, old memories fleeting between us. *Ask him*, I thought suddenly. *This is your chance.* He'd been there all along. Surely he knew something.

"One more question. And listen, I—I know this is weird. I'm sorry to ask you, but I just don't know who else would know. Did you ever meet my father?"

He paused, and then said carefully, "I didn't. She didn't tell anyone who he was. She was very clear that she didn't want any of us to know. Your mother is a very private woman."

There was a silence.

"Do you know, then," I asked quietly, "what we've been living on all this time?"

He studied the floor, hands clasped, shifted, and scratched his beard uncomfortably. "Well. So. You know she worked at a law firm. A prestigious one, I believe. But she got . . . well. She became erratic. She stopped going into the office. And they let her go, and she—you know your mother. There was a settlement."

This could be one big question answered. We could be living on the payout of her illness, the last vestiges of her normal life, when she had dressed in the morning, gone out to work, drunk coffee at a desk, asked for copies from a legal assistant. If it was true, she had stretched out that payment for years upon years, raising a child, alone, in a ruinously expensive city. She had bought a Yorkville apartment with it. She had paid for rent on the Ninety-Sixth Street place and my clothes and food and movie tickets and—

—no. That didn't add up. This was a piece of the puzzle, maybe, but not the whole thing.

I thanked Jim and clung to him when I hugged him goodbye. "You're looking well," he said gruffly, and turned the three familiar deadbolts on his door behind me.

I went home to Tor's apartment and let Mischief out of her carrier with a sigh of relief. She hopped up in my lap, and I started doing some mental addition. We had spent a few summers in my old nanny Margaret's tiny apartment, empty during her trips back to Hungary, while Mom sublet to summer associates at the city's white-shoe law firms. Every August we returned to an apartment fairly wrecked by entitled shit-head law students, vomit on the curtains, dings on the walls, and weeks of trash blocking the back door. She had just started renting out my room in the Upper West Side apartment during the year, but rent-stabilized leases only allow you to charge portions of the rent commensurate to the square footage; you can't profit off taking in roommates or subtenants. So where was the money coming from?

Or from whom?

Tor kept the dog. He discovered that if she were locked in the bedroom, she would sleep contentedly through the day.

I got on the plane to London and tried to be someone else for a year. I lived in a bunker-like dorm on the grounds of the university's medical school, and the other students on my floor came home each evening stinking of the formaldehyde from the corpses they were dissecting. I got a job in a pub. I had never had a drink, and on my first day, I tried to make a bemused patron a gin and tonic in a pint glass. Having wrangled an open long-distance relationship with Tor, I dated a tall, lanky guy in my creative writing class, who wrote me love poems referencing Norse mythology and liked to wear skirts in bed. I asked out my Tintin-doppelganger history professor, who was (obviously, in retrospect) gay, and who let down the foolish American as nicely as he could. I went to a lot of concerts and took a lot of walks and skipped a lot of classes and drank a lot of beer. I was pretty thrilled to have an identity that was "foreign/American" rather than "hopelessly weird," and that shift was one of the first cracks that let in the light that Leonard Cohen promised.

When I came back from England, twenty pounds heavier—while working for £3 an hour, I took to living, like the rest of the bar staff, on the leftover fries that came back on the pub patrons' plates—and cranky from missing London, Mom took back the dog promptly, sure that would convince me to move back in with her. (It didn't.) But we made up, tentatively, and saw each other a few times after I returned.

One night right before I went back to college, over dinner at her favorite restaurant, she got tipsy on a single glass of wine. She leaned across the table and said, abruptly: "You don't think I *really* went without sex all these years, do you?"

I spluttered. Why were we discussing sex over dumplings? I had never questioned why my mother didn't date. Her story when I was very young was that most molested children are abused by their stepfathers or the boyfriends of their mothers, and she didn't want to put me in danger. Later, she hardly left her room; where or how would she meet someone?

But apparently she had. She had been dating someone—a man she referred to coyly as "Mr. X," like we were starring in some weird post-Soviet thriller—since I was a toddler. Since, as you'll recall, she'd been married to her second, absent, abusive, now-dead husband. For almost two decades, all while we were living in the same apartment and sleeping in adjoining bedrooms. (I feel this is worth repeating, because how, *how*.)

"But—I don't understand," I finally got out. "Why was it a secret?"

She rolled her eyes as if amazed that anyone could be so dense. "*Elizabeth*. He's not . . ." She paused delicately, casting her eyes up for the right phrasing. ". . . free."

And I thought about the long-forgotten voices in the hallway as Brian/Billy sprinted for the bathroom, and her zero-to-sixty rage, and the fear that spurred it.

She wasn't angry because I'd been making out with my boyfriend. She was terrified because she'd almost gotten caught.

Until then, I thought I had a handle on what might be a lie and what wasn't. I thought I knew *this* subset of things to be true, as distinct from *that*; I knew about things that had really happened because I saw them with my own eyes. Because I was there.

But I had been there all along, and I didn't know that there was someone else in my mother's orbit. I didn't know that there was someone in my apartment during the long hours when I was at school, someone opening the fridge door to rummage among the soda cans, or idly running his hand over the spines of the books that lined our hallways. In my room, maybe, using the second bathroom; pushing past my coat to hang up his own. At night, the homework and Chinese food, the viewings of *Wild America* and *America's Funniest Home Videos*. During the day, a tall, male, half-dressed secret.

The building staff must have known, the doormen who verified every visitor by intercom. They would have seen him leave at lunchtime, then silently watched my mother bring me back home in the late afternoon, skipping, sticky with ice cream from the Sedutto's down the street. We were hot-bedding the same apartment, he and I, taking shifts in the task of providing companionship to my mother. Key difference, though: he knew about me, and I didn't know about him.

All these lies made me feel like a subpar oceanographer. I clung to my radar and my instruments, plotting the exact point of every tinge of sincerity, every note that rang true. She had constructed a new story for herself, making everything come out all right, everyone live happily ever after, starring herself as the heroine who raised me up from seed and myself as the miracle child with a great destiny ahead. That was the story she told everyone, including me. But I didn't believe it, not anymore. And so I was left searching for those elusive whales of truth, heaving under the surface.

We sat across the table from each other, trying to think of something to say. I didn't know how to reach the truth without sending the whales snorting and blowing out of the reach of my ship. If I had missed twenty years of an affair happening ten feet from my bedroom, what else didn't I know?

I shut my mouth and reached for the last of the soy sauce.

Later that year, I put the rest of the pieces together. I was at the office of her childhood friend, a laconic man who had hovered at the very periphery of my life as a bat mitzvah guest and an occasional voice on the other end of the phone. He was giving me a ready-to-be-discarded printer from his office. As I backed carefully down the hallway holding my end, a friend conscripted into service gamely steering with the other, I opened my mouth to ask about the email address he had used to send me directions, an unusual nickname, maybe—Basher T.? Why Basher?—and the letters swam and the emphasis rearranged itself. Not Basher, no initial T. The Hebrew word *bashert*: a soulmate, a match made literally in heaven.

I stumbled and nearly dropped the printer. My friend cursed, steadied the edge on his knee. I gripped harder, avoided his eyes as I backed up. Mr. X was married. Of course he was married. *Of course*. He had two daughters, one my age. I hope to God my mother was never in their house; too many refracted lives lived in too many small spaces. Too many chemtrails of lies.

They kept the affair a secret for twenty years, but his wife eventually found out. They divorced, and he moved to California, remarried and disappeared from my mother's life. My mother dated another old friend, a recent widower, but gave it up out of boredom. She had started putting on substantial weight—a petite woman who weighed two digits when she got pregnant with me, she was now well past two hundred pounds—and she went from rarely leaving the building to rarely leaving her bedroom, tucked up in bed watching the talking-heads political shows and eating Hershey's bars by the six-pack. Didn't she want to try auditing another class at her beloved Barnard? I asked. She had taken a class about the novel with Mary Gordon, and sat in the first row with a group of fellow feisty, elderly alums; it was one of the best years of her life. No, she waved me away; too much effort.

One day, in a maudlin mood, she asked me to "ask Google" where Mr. X was; I found his obituary.

She wept. She was at the age when more often than not, news of a friend was more likely to be a death than a move, a retirement, a new grandchild. I felt for her loss, but also thought, uneasily, that her grief was somehow overstepping into a role that wasn't hers. The time she spent with him was time taken away from his real family, his wife and children. She never talked about him with me after that first revelation, and I don't know exactly what she got from that relationship—whether it was love, or joy, or a reminder that she was still a full person and not just a full-time mother. Maybe it was no more than a way to pass the time, to fill the stretches of unaccounted-for hours from drop-off to pickup. Maybe he gave her the feeling of being a real and whole person, a feeling that with two small children of my own, I sympathize with. On many days, he must have been the only adult she spoke to.

And maybe it was more mercenary than that. Maybe this was the rest of the story that Jim didn't know. Maybe he was giving her money. Maybe this was the secret benefactor who had kept us housed and fed and entertained. Not an exchange for sex, nothing so crass, but a gift from an old friend, charity from someone who could work—who could function in the world—to a loved one who couldn't. By then I certainly knew a little something about how he might have felt.

CHAPTER 5

Launched

The year I was born, Jackie Kennedy Onassis was working as an editor at Doubleday. I like to imagine that she sat down at a formidable dark-wood desk every morning, crisply dressed, and worked her way through manuscripts in silence, marking them up with a blue pencil, and that every afternoon at five p.m. her assistant knocked on her office door bearing a glass of perfectly chilled chardonnay.

Publishing was no longer quite so glamorous by the time I showed up. Neither, in fairness, was I.

I had interned at the merged Bantam Doubleday Dell in high school. I worked for a subsidiary rights coordinator and spent most of my time editing down cover copy into smaller and simpler segments, suitable for non-native English-speaking agents and scouts, for the rights guide. Twice a week after my last class ended, I took the subway to Times Square, hunkered down in an unused storeroom qua office, and typed happily away. I was really in it for the book room: a bedroom-sized storage closet, crammed with metal shelving set in narrow aisles, with extra copies of books jammed in every which way. "Take whatever you want from there," said my frazzled supervisor as she rushed by. She didn't have to tell me twice. BDD published genre fiction, and piles of it. I stocked up on my beloved science fiction, piles of paperbacks with gleaming robots and ringed planets crowding the covers. I piled up new fiction in hardcover—Hardcover! Unimaginable luxury!—and squirreled everything away in my bedroom. The next year, I passed that internship along to my camp friend Arie with tips on which managers to ask for interesting work, and painstakingly described directions from the elevator to the book room. No fool he, he came prepared with an empty backpack.

I got my first job out of college at Bantam Dell, which had just cut off Doubleday as a stand-alone imprint, on a different floor of the same building. We shared the building with BMG, and every now and then as you passed the cargo entrance, a giant garage door would roll up and a limousine would glide smoothly out. Once, I caught a glimpse of Michael Jackson's drained face and tousled hair as the window rolled up. We loved those celebrity sightings but thought of them as taking place in another world; as entertainment went, books were the slim-margin, grubby, ink-stained stepchild to the real work of the building.

I worked for a gorgeous, energetic romance editor named Kara, only a few years older than I was. She'd picked me out of a pile of equally eager, equally unqualified bright-eyed, bushy-tailed English majors because "I saw you used to work in a bar, and I figured you'd be fun." We quickly became friends and went out to author lunches and book parties as often as

I could convince her to take me along. Her mother, a fierce, tiny Italian woman from Scranton, would call multiple times a day with questions and commentary; once, I had to stick my burning face into Kara's office and say, "Listen, I'm sorry, but she's asking—I would never ask otherwise but—OK, I'm just going to say it—your mom is in Banana Republic and wants to know what pants size you wear."

"Oh my Goooooood," she groaned. "Just transfer the call."

I knew it would be years before I was allowed to acquire any books of my own, and I was perfectly happy just being in proximity to books, typing up marketing plans, writing rejection letters, sending authors flowers on publication day. Once a month, the company ordered all the assistants pizza and we sat in a conference room for Slush Lunch, a beloved tradition where we opened all the unsolicited submissions we'd received from hopeful authors who hadn't managed to snag the attention of a literary agent. Most were just terrible, but there were enough doozies—prison mail (so much prison mail!), synopses scrawled in crayon, tinfoil-hat conspiracy theories, occasionally packaged in actual tinfoil—to keep us in material.

Romance writers like to have industry people speak at their conferences. Savvily, the southern chapters of the Romance Writers of America hold theirs in February. I made far too little money to take a proper vacation, but I spent many weeks in those first few winters holed up in janky Holiday Inn conference rooms during the day trying to look older than I was, and carousing drunkenly in the hotel pool at night with whatever assistant literary agent they'd brought down. The luxury of staying in a hotel—A hotel! In my own room!—just floored me. I shared a three-bedroom in Astoria with two beloved friends from summer camp, and I was grateful for the quiet.

Leaving for parts south also gave me some breathing room from my mother's increasingly frenzied calling. I didn't have a cell phone yet, and when I traveled I felt the lighthearted, childish glee of playing hooky; I was beyond where she could reach me. She raged upon every return—why hadn't I given her the number of the conference organizer or hotel security, what was *wrong* with me—but I was finally beginning to fully accept that her demands were bizarre and that I wasn't the problem. The boulder was off my chest. I still listened to the voice mails, tears of atavistic fear rushing to my eyes when she screamed, but I could also choose not to return them.

The fear wasn't entirely unwarranted. Something was changing with her. She was losing what little filter she'd had. My mother ran on pure vengeance, and age—hers or mine— hadn't slowed her down. When we fought, she would show up in the lobby of my office building, threatening security until they called me down. How a small woman with a heavy Queens accent managed to bully large, burly men into compliance, I don't know. But she did it. I would go down just to keep her from screaming the doors off. The last thing I needed was for my publisher to pass by and notice a resemblance. Far better to hustle her out the chrome revolving door, muttering apologies just to shut her up. I despaired of ever being fully out from under her thumb.

One spring evening, I was standing in a supermarket aisle debating the relative merits of two shapes of pasta when my brand-new Razr flip phone rang. I wedged it between my shoulder and ear. "Hello?"

The other end of the line was silent, and then there was

a sniffle. Then a keen. "Elizabeth . . ." Her voice trailed off. I groaned inwardly. It was Tranquilizer Voice.

"Hi, Mom. What's wrong?"

Another sniff. "Oh . . . you know. This is a hard time of year for me. I miss my mother, Elizabeth." Her mother was forty years dead, but every spring the grief came back as fresh as the first.

"I know, Mom. I'm sorry."

"I think she must be lonely, all by herself down there in her grave. Don't you think she must be *lonely*?"

I paused with the winning box of penne suspended above my basket. This was new.

"I. I mean. I don't think her soul is still there, Mom. I'm sorry, I know this is hard, but she's not in there anymore, you know? It's just her body."

That was a mistake. She wailed anew, and a woman walking by looked over her shoulder. I grimaced apologetically and turned toward the shelf with my shoulders hunched.

"Are you OK?"

"Well!" She seemed to gather herself. "I have an *idea*, Elizabeth. I think I know how we can fix this."

I did not like the sound of that "we."

"I know you don't want children. I know you don't. But, listen—hear me out. You could have a stillborn baby, right? You could do that."

I boggled, silently.

"And then—you see, this is brilliant! We could put the baby down in the grave with her, and she wouldn't be lonely. They would both have company. And everything would be alright." A beat passed, and she said, more gaily: "Well, just think about it. Think about it. Call me back."

She hung up, and I stared around the store with bugged-out eyes as other people went about their shopping, blissfully untroubled by the image of an arthritic elderly woman digging up her mother's grave by moonlight, a small bundle tucked under one arm.

I went home and opened a bottle of wine and watched *Buffy the Vampire Slayer* and tried to pretend that Joyce Summers was my mom. As coping mechanisms go, I highly recommend this.

As she got older, I liked to half-joke—gallows humor being a helpful crutch—that it was getting harder and harder to identify if any given act of shittiness was her dementia, her eccentricity, or just her being a garden-variety asshole. She had never had a firm hand on her temper, and with age she no longer seemed to even try to manage it, screaming red-faced at the slightest conversational hiccup. She also started to lose track of what she had done and when. An obsessively careful recordkeeper and the source of my habit of paying bills immediately when they arrived, she forgot to pay a $14 AmEx bill. When the next bill came with a late payment fee, she called the bank screaming furiously—How *dare* they, didn't they know her history as a stellar, upstanding customer?—and refused to pay the bill at all. The next month came with another fee, with a percentage of the whole charged as a penalty, and she threw it in a drawer. The next month came, and then the next. The bill rose more than a thousand dollars over that $14, and the credit card company called me, the rep's voice unctuous and faux-concerned—Didn't I want to pay her debt for her? Wasn't it the *right thing to do*?

I hung up on them.

Against the terms of her lease, she housed Columbia grad students and young office workers in the apartment's two extra bedrooms. They weren't allowed to have guests, and had to put up with her peculiarities, but for nominal rent in a twenty-four-hour doorman building half a block from Central Park, they paid up without a peep. Many of them were international students hungry for a connection of any kind, and years later, I am still in touch with many of them: the woman from East Germany who told me stories of life behind the Berlin Wall, her family of four sharing their four allotted bananas per year, grateful her father didn't like them so they could split his; the gay Argentine man who found New York much more libertine than Córdoba; the teacher from Istanbul who wrote to me in horror every time he saw a parallel between Trump and Erdoğan (he wrote often).

The bright side of her ever-slipping control was that she started telling me things she hadn't meant to. Most of them meant nothing: the names of men she'd dated in high school, trips she'd planned on taking. One afternoon she insisted on taking me out to lunch, and we sat at a sidewalk table outside a sushi restaurant. She puffed furiously while thumbing the menu. I had taken to buying her cartons of Marlboros from dubiously legal websites at cut-rate prices; the packages arrived weeks later stamped with customs marks from former Eastern Bloc countries. I hated being her supplier, but also knew things went better for me when she had nicotine to keep her calm.

"Ma'am," said the meek waitress, "I'm so sorry, but you can't smoke out—"

Mom turned her most terrifying gaze on her; the blue-steel barely-contained-rage glance over the bifocals. "Young *lady*," she bit out, "I have been smoking since before your mother failed to shut her legs for your father. And I don't intend to stop now. I want the tempura. Elizabeth?" She pointed her menu at me.

"Sushilunchspecialthankyou," I rushed out. Mom took my menu, slapped it together with hers, and handed the two over. The waitress caught my eye, and I mouthed *I am so, so sorry* as she backed away, shaking her head.

"Get *her*," Mom said cheerfully. "Telling *me* to stop smoking. Oh! I'm seeing that hypnotist again, though. He's helped me quit before."

"A *hypnotist*?" I said. "Like, with a pocket watch and a waistcoat?"

"No, no," she laughed, shaking her head. "He's a psychologist. You remember, I was seeing that David Kagan, but he gave up! He told me he couldn't do any more for me. Borderline isn't curable, he says. *I* think he's just lazy."

"Wait, what isn't curable?"

Her eyes flashed and she drew herself up. "Nothing. You mind your own business, Elizabeth. No one asked *you*."

Back at my desk, I looked it up: borderline personality disorder. At the opening words, "A mental health disorder . . . ," my head lit up, electric.

This wasn't just eccentricity. This was actual mental illness. BPD is a Cluster B personality disorder, usually the result of childhood trauma, which leaves the person permanently wavering between neurosis and psychosis. They often suffer from other mental illnesses and behavioral disorders, and find it difficult or impossible to regulate their emotions. They live with a paralyzing fear of abandonment, but an inability to maintain relationships. They're almost always women—the ones who get diagnosed, anyway. They're often mothers.

Who overreact.

Who compulsively manipulate.

Who are impulsive and paranoid.

Who lie and obscure.

Who cannot respect, or even bear the existence of, a boundary between themselves and their children.

Who view any disagreement as disloyalty, and lash out with violence.

So.

It had a name.

I was awash with relief. She wasn't just strict or difficult. She was dangerous. She was ill.

And it wasn't curable.

This knowledge made dealing with her rage no easier. But at least I knew, now, that the lifelong drumbeat in my head—*something is wrong here*—had been pounding out the truth. I wasn't being sensitive. I wasn't making it up. And the only effective approach was to withdraw. People suffering from borderline personality disorder live in a world on fire. The people in their lives are angels or demons, the best of friends or bitterest of enemies. The only expression of love in which my mother believed was the giving of all that I was, all of my time, all of my affection, all of my thoughts and feelings and secrets. If I failed to deliver everything to my mother, I'd failed, full stop. I'd abandoned her. There was no halfway mark. *Why don't you just call her less often*, well-meaning friends would ask, bewildered, and I would laugh disbelievingly.

It's impossible to understand the all-consuming wrath and love of someone suffering like this unless you've lived with it. My mother was the vortex of a hurricane, whose screaming winds and tons of swirling debris had only to touch me to sweep me up. The only way to avoid finding myself launched a mile above the earth was to stay the hell away.

✦ ✦ ✦

And so I retreated. I had plenty to distract me from the angry voice mails. I was hip-deep in a passionate relationship with my first girlfriend, made all the more dramatic by circumstance. Her mother was dying of a fast-growing brain tumor, and her plan to move across the country to seek her fortune in TV writing was put on hold until her mother died. When she wasn't at her mother's bedside, Caroline stayed in the Fifth Avenue apartment of a family friend, which was sitting vacant; the friend and his elderly mother spent their time at some undisclosed summer location. I had never seen anything like it. Dark, heavy furniture lined the rooms, and the "maid's room" behind the kitchen—unlike the one in my own apartment, which my mother rented out—had clearly been recently occupied by a real live maid. Ornate paneled walls met a meticulously painted ceiling. The dark furniture-oil smell of wealth permeated the rooms.

During those early days when we had sex all the time, every moment, making up for the years Caroline had spent in the closet, I spent a lot of time in that apartment. We slept on a pullout couch in the library, never touching the heavily furnished bedrooms. Political biographies and old VHS tapes lined the walls. When I left early in the morning, dressed in the same sales-rack office clothes I'd worn the day before, the doormen eyed me with more bemusement than mistrust. What was this shaggy creature doing in their lobby?

I had grown up barely a mile from that apartment, but a mile in New York can be a hundred thousand people and a handful of socioeconomic leaps. Caroline's old-money world was a world I didn't know. When navigating her aunt's cluttered apartment, I stumbled on a dusty book peeking out from under the coffee table; it was a *Who's Who*, a product I had previously believed to be an entirely fictional trope created for the benefit of romantic comedy scriptwriters, and Caroline had an entry in it. I laughed disbelievingly, and Caroline and her aunt looked at me puzzled; why wouldn't she? When her mother died, I was introduced ("my friend, Liz") to more than one person at the funeral with the surname Rockefeller. Her eternally disapproving father belonged to a social club. During her childhood they had summered (summered!) in Maine, where Caroline played tennis and basketball and carefully didn't look at the female lifeguards at the pool.

Here's what I learned about the very wealthy: they are regular, human people like you and me. But they are unencumbered by any notion of futility. Long after that funeral, when Caroline introduced me to her family and I got to know this bewildering group of anything-can-be-done pragmatists, Auntie asked me pointed questions about my family and where I had come from. She heard my story with a raised eyebrow and the furious demolition of one cigarette after another. "Little love," she growled. "This is not acceptable. Don't you want to know?"

"Know what?" I asked, mystified. "How? He's been dead for more than two decades. What could I know?"

"*Uch*. You have no imagination. Sweetheart, you need to find *out* about this man. Who was he? What was he like? What did he do? Do you have *grandparents* living?"

I didn't know the answer to any of these questions. I raised my hands helplessly, suddenly ashamed to have lost track of a whole side of my family in front of this pedigreed company.

She flicked an ash. "Let me see what I can do. What do you know about him?"

"I know his name."

She fixed steely blue eyes on me. "*And?*"

"And . . . he was blond, I think? And oh, I know how old he was. So probably his birth year?"

Auntie huffed. "Call your mother."

"Oh no, she doesn't talk about him. I can't—"

"Call. Your. Mother," she bit out.

And I did.

My voice shook as I got the words out. Caroline's aunt—yes, the rich one. The one who lived on Seventy-Ninth Street. She was offering to hire me a PI. This person would—no, I wasn't using drugs. What would a PI have anything to do with—no, I wasn't trying to talk over you, I just don't understand—OK. OK. I'm sorry. So the PI would be investigating Warren.

Warren Luther.

My father.

There was a silence.

"I'll see what I can remember," she said brusquely, and hung up.

An email arrived that night, uncharacteristically badly punctuated and abrupt.

Warren Frank Luther
8/18/49–10/2/77
520 E 81 St.
Parents Frank Luther and Dorothy Knox Luther

Sister???

(ex) wife Lydia Grant. Was attending law school. Don't know
    which one, or whether she ever graduated and practiced law.

Don't know whether she used married name.

Above is Lydia Grant's address. He had lost his job At American
    Express and moved in with her, perhaps. He had lived at 526
    E 82 St

Soc Sec # XXX XX XXXX

Cremated Garden State Crematory, North Bergen, NJ on Oct
    4, 1977. Don't know if ashes were interred.

Funeral Frank Campbell 1076 Madison Ave

Served in Viet Nam

I ticked off at least five new facts I knew about him now.
A veteran! My word. Someone's brother. With . . . family in
New Jersey? Maybe? I was more flummoxed about the facts
my mother knew. If they had really dated for so short a time,
why on earth did she know his Social Security number? What
tabs had she been keeping? Where were the records?

I thought of the dull-green file cabinet in her closet, locked
up tight. I'd been right. Somewhere in there was everything
I wanted to know. There was no pushing her—she'd keep
doling out tidbits once every few years until either she took
enough of her tranquilizers to spout it all out, or I went over
there with a baseball bat and smashed the lock.

The baseball bat sounded better, frankly.

I shuffled the facts in her email into something resembling
a narrative for the PI, apologizing for not knowing more. I
cringed at how it all looked, so tawdry, so irresponsible, to
know so little about my own father. I settled down to wait for
as long as it took to dig out my life's long mystery.

Two days later, my desk phone rang. "Little love, it's Auntie. We're on a conference call with Mr. Jacobson and he's got some information on your dad."

I sat in a row of low-walled cubicles that ran down the middle of the Bantam Dell hallway, like a lackey moat that kept the more junior editors (interior offices) from ousting the more senior editors (window offices). In practice, this meant that people streamed past me on both sides all day long. I hunched down in my chair and tried to create a soundproof booth with my shoulders.

The PI was calm and just-the-facts—surreally so, given how hard my heart was thumping in my chest. He had the name and a phone number for Warren's ex-wife. He also had the phone number for my aunt—my *aunt*—who lived on Roosevelt Island with my uncle and cousins. He paused when he came to the names of my grandparents—who were, I now discovered, long dead—and his businesslike tone suddenly warmed.

"*Oh!*" he said. "Frank Luther! Goodness, I know who that is. He was a children's entertainer when I was a kid. I listened to him on the radio all the time. Isn't that something?"

Indeed, it was—something.

I asked Auntie how much it had cost so that I could reimburse her. She told me without hesitation that it was fifty dollars, and I wrote her a check, my hand slow so my appalling handwriting would come out more respectably. It wasn't until years later that I realized it had certainly cost more, much more, and that she had just made up an amount she thought I could afford. The ironic part was, I barely could.

I called the ex-wife first. A matter-of-fact voice on the other end of the phone informed me that she had never heard of a Warren Luther and certainly had never been married to one, sorry she couldn't help. I hung up the phone ready to throttle someone, anyone, with frustration. I had no way of knowing if the woman was telling the truth. Her name was a common one, and the PI could have had the wrong person. The real ex-wife could have taken and kept Warren's name, or remarried and taken yet a third. Or the woman on the phone could have wanted no part of this surprise offspring, and have gotten rid of me as briskly as dusting off her hands. I had no idea how to ferret out the truth.

On to the sister.

Helen and her husband lived on Roosevelt Island, a narrow strip of land in the East River built up with apartment buildings and a few small stores. A winding road leads to a historical district containing an abandoned smallpox hospital, and to the Octagon, the last vestige of the former New York City Lunatic Asylum. My childhood friend Gretchen lived in Helen's building and knew her daughter. Worlds collided again: Had my cousin and I unknowingly attended the same birthday parties, splashed together in the community pool, watched Fourth of July fireworks over the East River from the same flotilla of folding chairs?

I barricaded myself in an empty conference room and called her husband at his office, hoping to start with someone less emotionally involved. He was taken aback; whether he'd ever met Warren I don't know, but he was a husband, and he was thinking of his wife. He agreed hesitantly to put us in touch, and that evening I dialed their home number with my heart in my throat.

He had prepared her for the call. It must have felt like the world's worst boomerang, like a dead hand reaching out from a grave long settled. Warren had caused his family so much grief, had killed himself in the messiest, most public way imaginable. But here out of nothingness was his child. Her niece. The product of a relationship with a woman whose name they'd never heard. Twenty-five years down the line, he was still scattering stones in her path.

I thought she might be worried that I was looking for money, hoping to cash in on some kind of Dead-Dad Jackpot. I had no proof that I was his daughter, only a timeline and possibly a resemblance. My mother had kept no pictures, or no pictures she would admit to; the best I had was an Oldsmobile ad she had ripped from a magazine circa 1978, when she knew she was pregnant and was trying to figure out how to describe to future-me what he looked like. A soft-focus young man stands in a crowd behind a car, all of them in tennis whites. He looks about as much like Warren as any blond Caucasian man looks like another—70s haircut, far-off expression.

"Hello?" said a careful, New York City–accented voice on the other end of the phone. (We do have accents! We do! We just sound so much like anchorpeople that you can't tell.)

"H-hello," I stuttered out. "Um. Helen Cooper?"

"Yes. You must be Liz."

"Yes, I—sorry. I have no idea what to say here." I giggled nervously; there was no return sympathy laugh. "I think your brother, Warren, was my father, and I just—I was hoping to talk to someone who had known him."

A beat, and then a sigh. "I'll try and help, Liz. But you should understand that it's been a long time, and my brother and I did not get along. I'm not sure how much I can tell you."

She was true to her word. Five minutes of largely monosyllabic answers and an extracted promise to send a picture later, we hung up. Our stilted conversation left me with a hole in the bottom of my stomach. I had been prepared for a grieving sister, or a joyful aunt, or a confused version of either. What I hadn't expected was a woman who sounded like she just plain hadn't liked her brother, and who had never thought that he might show up in her life again. She didn't want to talk about him, and she didn't want to talk to me. She was kind enough, but the idea that we'd have some kind of sweet belated reunion clearly had been wishful thinking. I realized with a sinking heart that the fact that I'd built him into a hero in my head did not mean that he'd been a good guy, or an uncomplicated one. His own nearest relative sure wasn't a fan. I had no idea why. But one more door had closed.

I was closer, but still not close enough. I had some bullet points about him, which was much more than I'd had before. But I had no stories. There was no color to him. I was fixated on at least knowing what he'd looked like. If I had a picture, I thought, I could look at his eyes and try to suss out what was behind them. I could try to read humor or sadness or frustration or boredom in his expression. Some amount of photographic forensics could be performed. I was sure of it.

And so I waited. Every night, I came home from work with my heart in my throat, dashing for the kitchen table where my roommates and I threw the mail, looking for an envelope.

I didn't hear from her for a year and a half.

Why hasn't she *sent* it, I lamented to everyone I saw. How long could it take to find a picture? How long could it take to send? Couldn't she hear in my voice how much I needed this, how desperate I was? Didn't she care?

It's a hard lesson that when your need bumps up against a stranger's pain, their pain always takes precedence. I wasn't even a bit player in her story; maybe, I reasoned, she was hoping I would just go away if ignored. What is she *doing*, I keened to Guylaine, my Québécoise girlfriend, who had just moved to New York to give our relationship a try. (Caroline was long gone to LA to make a career out of writing for TV.) Older, wiser, and conversant in the language of grief, she counseled patience, and warned that I should make my peace with the possibility that I would never hear from Helen again.

Ha *ha*. It's like she'd never met me. I had twenty-five years of pent-up wondering in the hopper, and I was *thisclose* to finding out what he looked like. Patience my *ass*.

When I couldn't bear it anymore—eighteen months of adrenaline swamping the system every time key hit lock was too much—I wrote her a letter. It is, thank God, lost to history. I'm sure it was histrionic. I know I begged her. I told her how big and empty the hole was that Warren had left, and how much a picture would mean to me, and how I would never contact her again if that was what she wanted, just please: show me his face.

It doesn't often snow in New York. The heat from the densely set buildings rises, and the snow turns to rain before it hits the pavement. But it was blizzarding for real the day I walked into my kitchen with Guylaine, laughing over some story she'd told me about her students. We stomped snow off our boots, and I undid the toggles on my ludicrously insufficient suede coat with embroidery down the front, which I had bought on clearance at Loehmann's (RIP) and of which I was inordinately proud.

The pile of mail had a Christmas card on top, with a red envelope and dove-bearing-holly-sprig stamp, which was unusual for my all-Jewish household. Frowning, I flipped it over and looked at the return address.

Cooper. Roosevelt Island.

I sat down with a *whoomph*, right onto the kitchen floor. Guylaine squatted down beside me. "Babe! What on earth . . . ?"

I slit open the envelope with one shaking finger. The card fell into my lap, spilling a handful of faded square photographs.

The card was brief. They were all the pictures she could find of her brother. She wished me a merry Christmas.

The pictures showed a young blond man in a succession of soft, too-big button-down shirts. They were taken in what appears to be a Manhattan apartment much like mine looked in the 70s: olive-green curtains, a squat rotary phone, burnt-orange carpet, a bookshelf full of vinyl records. In one, an older man in a dapper suit, with a deep widow's peak and an exquisite handlebar mustache, demonstrates a plastic toy for a blond toddler as a late-twenties Warren looks fondly on. In another, Warren sits on a couch with a well-dressed woman with a white Betty Ford pouf who is holding balloons for the same toddler, smiling brightly, a glass of what might be sangria by her side.

In the days that followed, everyone who saw those pictures—and I thrust them into the hands of everyone I knew, *This is him, this is my father, I think it's him. Do you see a resemblance? Do you think I look like him?*—asked if it was me in the striped romper, with the short hair and the wide smile. If that was me in the bib, carefully stroking Warren's stubble, if that was me in his arms, grinning up at him as he looks down solemnly, protectively, into my face.

It's not. It's another small child of his acquaintance, probably his nephew—my cousin!—James. By the time I was that age, he was already long dead.

Guylaine studied the pictures over my shoulder, her breath warm on my neck. "A good-looking man," she said reflectively.

"He is," I said. "He was."

I sent Helen the biggest bouquet I could afford, with an effusive note of thanks. I never heard from her again.

But every once in a while I looked up her daughter, Jenna, Gretchen's friend, on Facebook. I don't know what I was looking for; she was hardly going to post an impromptu treatise about long-lost relatives and how great they are, and about how pleased she'd be if any reached out to her. She looked nothing like me, and of course she wouldn't. Her mother was adopted, my mother thought she remembered, and if so we weren't related by blood. But I kept peering at her thumbnail profile photo regardless, trying to make her features come into focus, trying to make her familiar. I wanted her to look like family. I kept trying to work up the courage to reach out.

(Twenty years later, one housebound day during the early weeks of COVID-19 lockdown, I idly looked her up and found her obituary. Shocked, I texted Gretchen, chilled that Jenna too might have killed herself; she was only forty-two. But no. Heart attack. Helen was mourning yet another loss, one she couldn't even dignify with an in-person funeral.

And I had missed my chance to look my cousin in the eye.)

I stalled out with that envelope in hand. I thought the pictures would be enough. They *were* enough, for a long time. Fitting a face—even a static one from an old photograph—onto the image I'd pieced together, uncomfortably, like a kid's rubber Halloween mask onto a dress form, was enough information to stun me. I moved through that next month in a fog.

I scanned the photos on the office scanner and emailed them to friends across the world; this was before cloud drives were a thing, and now that I had the photos I feared losing them, fiercely. I framed the one of him holding the inquisitive toddler and put it on my dresser.

Is that you?

No.

I did some desultory research. I googled his name. I looked up birth and death records. There was nothing out there; since he died young, many years before the internet existed, there was very little online record of him. I ordered the DVD of my grandfather crooning his way through *High Hat*. So charming, but one step removed from the man I was searching for.

The PI had turned up new details, and I followed them up. Warren's funeral had been held at the famous Upper East Side funeral home Frank E. Campbell, which has hosted the funerals of every wealthy person you could think of: Rudolph Valentino, Tennessee Williams, Leona Helmsley, Ayn Rand, the Notorious B.I.G. And, apparently, Warren Luther. It was across the street from my elementary school, because of course it was. I ducked in one day, unplanned; I had to surprise myself, or I would have lost my nerve. I explained myself to the woman at reception, and she sent me to the director, an appropriately solemn man behind a heavy, impressive desk. He clasped his hands and regarded me solemnly.

"Young lady, I'm sorry; it must be very sad not to have a burial place to visit. Let's see what I can do to help you. Let's get some information." He took out a notebook and a weighty pen, started a fresh page. "Name?"

"Warren Luther. Frank. I mean, Warren Frank Luther."

"Date of death?"

I told him.

"Date of birth?"

I floundered, forgetting in the moment that it had been in

my mother's email. "I'm sorry. I don't know. He would have been in his late twenties."

"Ah." He peered at me. "Well, documentation would be your friend here. Do you have a copy of your parents' marriage certificate? That would have it."

"Oh, they weren't married," I said. "But I'm sure I can find out—"

At the words "weren't married," the director closed his notebook and sat back. "I'm sorry, Miss," he said, not unkindly. "I'm afraid I don't know that we can be of any help to you."

Surely I had misunderstood; surely I had not stepped into some kind of Eisenhower-era biopic. It was the twenty-first century. Surely this man was not mentally branding me with a scarlet B. His eyes were steady on me, his face friendly but shuttered. My eyes pricked with tears. I stood up from the chair that cost more than my rent, painfully aware of my H&M blazer and Jewish nose. "Thank you," I said blindly, and fled.

The crematorium was no more help. The very kind voice on the other side of the phone luckily did not seem to care about the marital status of my erstwhile parents, but she had only the handwritten paperwork, in which someone had picked up the ashes and signed an illegible scribble, likely Lydia. There was no indication that they had been interred anywhere, meaning they could have been scattered off the prow of a ship or buried in someone's backyard, or could be sitting in a breakfront somewhere in a peppy floral tin, like the remains of my childhood dog. There would be no cinematic graveside visit. The trail was cold.

And so I sat on it. One victory and one failure had sapped my momentum. I hung the photos around my bedroom, my fingerprints permanently oiled into the frames where I held them up to my face, trying to ferret out what he had been thinking or feeling, ticking off every similarity. That soft-focus face, the familiar details of nose and smile and cowlick, the unfamiliar assembly of the whole, was all I could handle. I was full, just short of choking. It took a long time to settle.

My days were too busy for much self-searching, anyway. I had graduated with $30,000 in student debt, a sum that now seems paltry next to the six figures that my lawyer and doctor friends live with, but it was as much as my starting salary. I doubtfully began paying my $175.46 a month, my payoff date so far in the future it might as well be science fiction. I was making the bills by cobbling together a handful of short-term jobs—data entry, catering, book reviews—on top of my full-time one, but I was only just coming out even every month.

And then Mom called, panicking, her voice shrill. All I could understand were the words "homeless shelter" over and over.

She had fallen behind on the rent, and the landlord had started eviction proceedings.

CHAPTER 6

Selling for Scrap

The waiting room of the Center for Women's Reproductive Care at Columbia was nice enough, as waiting rooms go. It had bland but pleasant beige décor, pastel chairs, inoffensive prints of soothing landscapes. The receptionists were efficient and kindly; they were used to dealing with women who were not only under a great deal of pressure, but also on a whole lot of hormones.

I didn't plan to have children. Put more accurately: I planned to have no children. Maternal instinct had skipped right over me. Women in New York don't breed young. When I started a job in the Midwest in my midthirties and found that several colleagues my own age were already grandmothers, a fact no one found particularly noteworthy, I had to clench my teeth to keep my jaw from hitting my chest. At twenty-five, no one I knew was in spitting distance of thinking about considering maybe possibly someday talking about having kids. Least of all me.

If you've ever been on a college campus, or on a bus or a subway, or flipped idly to the back of a magazine, you've seen the ads. A soft-focus young woman smiles into the middle distance, or cradles a flower lovingly in her hands. "Give the gift of life!" the copy trumpets. "Help create a family!" "We're looking for angels!"

I fell for these ads, hard. I won't tell you I "donated" eggs out of altruism. I could no more have fully comprehended the pain of infertility than I could have flapped my arms and flown to the moon. But I was still working as an assistant editor, and the $8,000 compensation for egg donation was three months' salary. Even without the eviction notice, that would have been a dizzyingly seductive amount. Every month I balanced my checkbook and noted with a sinking heart how little I was able to save after bills and student loans. What would I do when I started having to fully support my mother as well, rather than just sending checks here and there? And how, while we're thinking about it, would I come up with retirement savings so that I didn't become her forty years down the line?

The monetary aspect did give me some pause. It felt unnervingly like selling children. The ads (which I didn't yet know are often shameless bait-and-switches) offer higher prices to donors with Ivy League degrees, or with certain ethnic make-ups, or who are, say, over a certain height. It felt off-putting to put a dollar value on those things.

I was naive. I had no idea how many dozens of hours I would end up cooling my heels in the waiting room with other ragged-at-the-edges, slightly shamed-looking young women. After taxes, all the morning waiting, the shots, and the surgery itself, the per-hour money whittled away pretty quickly. When I started taking meds for the thyroid disorder that has been linked with the high doses of Lupron I was given—a drug then used in donor protocols at high daily doses, off label—the copays took care of the rest. Which is not to say it wasn't worth it. That $5,000 after taxes did provide an emotional barrier between me and the fear of running out of money, but it was compensation for time spent not doing other paid work, not a windfall.

Knowing I couldn't trust my own valuation of fertility—pregnancy seemed like something people would pay to avoid, rather than mortgage the house to achieve—I listened to the clinic's shtick. "Egg donation *saves lives*," the coordinator told me earnestly, holding my gaze. "Infertility is so destructive that it's correlated with suicide. You could be saving a life as well as creating one!" I nodded uncertainly. "You're a *hero*," she said.

I didn't feel like a hero. I felt like a product. The family history form they gave me to fill out was dozens of pages long and intimidatingly in-depth. It asked for complete medical histories on both sides, my own medical history, academics, interests, hobbies, athletics. I dug way back in my memory to remember my SAT scores and what extracurriculars I'd done in high school, so the clinic could try to make a match.

It wasn't until after I was chosen by the first set of recipients that I started to understand the full desperation of the women and couples going through this process. In some respects I must have looked like a good selection—tall, blond, thin, Seven Sisters education, gainfully employed. But who looked at my family's medical history—my mother's cornucopia of medical woes, my father's blank page ("cause of death: suicide; medical history: unknown") and thought, *Boy, this horse'll run?*

Only someone for whom this is the last resort.

The protocol I was on is, thankfully, rarely used now. For

many weeks, I took Lupron every day to decrease my hormonal load and stop ovulation. Essentially, I was turning my uterus into a balloon—an empty sack with a thin lining, ready to grow the super-follicles for retrieval. In large doses, Lupron throws your hormones entirely out of whack; it's now used as a puberty blocker for gender-confirmation therapy in teenagers. They started me off at the highest dose, twenty units every day, and for those first weeks I woke up every hour during the night, soaked in sweat and radiating heat.

I couldn't wrap my head around the idea of giving myself an injection. I can't have been the only one, as the clinic held a donor injection class. This was the only time in this regimented, rigidly anonymized process when I could reliably identify other women as donors, and all these years later, I still remember their faces. Any thoughts I'd had about baby engineering were confirmed in an instant. I had some assumptions about the recipients. They were likely to be wealthy—the average cost of donor-egg IVF in the early 2000s was in the five digits, after insurance—and therefore, our world being what it is, were likely to be white. Otherwise, though, I expected the regular mix of wealthy-and-white—different hair colors, heights, weights, features. And if you were going through all the pain, the effort, the cost, the night sweats, and the risk of failure and ensuing heartbreak to have a pregnancy, if you were going to try to pass the child off as the product of your own DNA, wouldn't you try to have a child who looked like you?

Apparently not. Every donor in that room was tall, blond, and skinny. I had just finished a marathon, and was five foot eight and 130 pounds—the lightest I had ever been in my adult life—and I visibly outweighed the other women there. Unless this was an extraordinary coincidence in which each of our recipients happened to fit the same profile, these women were hand-selecting—from vital stats, not even pictures—source material they thought might give their children an edge.

We practiced injections on oranges, and on fist-sized fake butts. Somewhere out there, some put-upon brand manager at a pharmaceutical company had hit upon the idea of creating silicone butts with the name of a drug emblazoned on one cheek. We snickered, we squinted, and we stabbed, badly. I felt like I was failing at decorating a very tiny cake.

They waited to give me the check until after the retrieval—I guess to avoid me running off with my check and my grapefruit-sized ovaries and my needle-pockmarked stomach without going through the final step. I woke up in recovery to find the check sitting on my blanketed lap, and looked at the nurses surreptitiously to see if any of them were judging me for anything I may have said under the influence of the anesthesia. A nurse came around, relieved me of my blanket, let in my friend who had come to pick me up, and ushered us through the back door and down the cargo elevator, away from the eyes of the real patients sitting in the waiting room. I scurried out into the bright light of Midtown, still a little woozy, and not a little unnerved by the fact that a doctor had just put a large needle into my vagina and extracted a bunch of eggs.

Installed safely on my couch and chugging Gatorade to stave off ovarian hyperstimulation syndrome, I tried to come to terms with what had just happened. Somewhere out there, a woman was about to be pregnant, maybe, with a baby that was made from my DNA. The recipients knew everything about me except my face and my name, but all I knew about them was that they could afford—or could borrow enough to afford—the procedure. Better than most, I knew that just wanting a baby isn't enough. Neither is love. What, I thought sickly, if I had just delivered a baby into a house like mine?

Commercial DNA tests were still years in the future, and the clinic's message to donors was clear: Stay out of it. Let the parents keep the secret. If the kids find out about you, the lie will be exposed, and the family will be destroyed. You don't want to destroy a family, now do you?

I didn't. But I had an inkling that something wasn't right with that argument. Not knowing my father had been an enormous hole in my life. Hadn't I just done the same thing to someone else? How could I justify it?

I couldn't. At all. But I rationalized. I didn't want to raise children, but having my genes in the world seemed like it might be OK. I knew what it was like to grow up under the weighted blanket of the wrong kind of love. If I had kids myself, I might end up exactly like my mother. The only safe place for my kids to be might be somewhere else. I still wrestled with guilt, but I tried to put stats around that fear: most houses are solid, most parents are not abusive, most kids are fine. I hoped.

I had lunch with Janet, a writer I had been working with for some time—a cheerful, no-nonsense career author with an adored eight-year-old daughter. We sat at a two-top at an outdoor café, and she told me all about the little girl—her hobbies, her sports, and her school. And, unexpectedly, her donor mom. My heart tightened painfully.

"Well," I said, "I haven't told anyone else in our field this, but I was a donor this year. I've felt kind of guilty about—"

And I got no further, because she had pushed our sandwiches to the side, hurled herself across the table, slung her arms around my neck, and started crying. "*Thank you*," she wept into my neck. "Thank you for doing that."

This was a human face on what I'd only seen as a simple mathematical equation. I had good eggs, some women had none; I had blood and plasma, someone needed it; years later, a friend had zero working kidneys, I had two. But Janet's tears gave me hope. If she was good to her kid, maybe this was the norm. Maybe I hadn't engaged in some kind of prenatal human trafficking. Maybe I'd done something good after all. Maybe I'd found a way to have children that wouldn't involve wrecking them.

So when the clinic called back, I answered. And a third time. Multiple births from IVF were then not uncommon. I now have between zero and nine genetic children running around—more, if the recipient couple adopted out leftover embryos—ranging in age from around thirteen to sixteen. But by the fourth time they called, I was sore—carrying around giant ovaries for too long is tiring and uncomfortable, and I had abdominal pain that my gynecologist thought might come from internal scarring. I was done.

The clinic got pushy, buoying up my suspicion that the donations had been successful. I was making them money and upping their success stats. This did not make me particularly amenable to the high-pressure guilt act they put on. The language around altruism suddenly came back: Didn't I *want* to help an infertile couple? Wasn't I willing to *do the work*? I did not say any of the things I was thinking, as I was not raised in a barn. But I thought them. Loudly.

I left my contact information with the clinic in case the children wanted to contact me. They looked at me doubtfully and put a Post-it in the file. I thought a lot about what would happen if the children and I ever met. Would they look familiar to me, or I to them? Would we have anything to talk about, anything in common? Would they be angry with me for "giving them up" in the way that an adopted child might be angry with a birth mother? Would they want a relationship, or just a medical history? Would they have wondered about me, as I wondered about them?

I was twenty-eight when I did my third and last donation, the same age as Warren when he died. I'm not superstitious, but that was the year I looked both ways extra carefully when crossing the street. When my birthday rolled around I breathed a sigh of relief, feeling like I'd put one over on the universe—like I'd pulled the handle and gotten three cherries in a row and *ding ding ding*: special bonus years. I went one way, and my possible offspring another. For now.

❖ ❖ ❖

I hired a lawyer and paid my mother's back rent. With the landlord mollified and a narrow margin of error padding my bank account, I began to relax. Crisis averted for the time being. The $30K I was making, minus taxes, plus four part-time gigs, covered the $600 a month I paid for my third of the rent. It also covered my bills, a few bills of my mother's, the cost of enough beer to try and largely fail to pick up women, and a retirement account where I stashed every other penny. It made me feel safe. Like *fuck*, I thought, was I going to end up like my mother.

I cut my hair off and dyed it peroxide blond, with an effect decidedly more preppy than punk. I looked like a prefect at Eton, minus the white tie. I didn't tell anyone at work that I was dating women. I didn't feel like it would go over so well in the universally hetero world of early 2000s romance publishing. They'd all met Torsten when I started work, and I just kind of failed to mention that we broke up shortly thereafter.

They were decent people and probably, in retrospect, wouldn't have cared. But I felt like I finally had a chance to fade into the background, and I grabbed it tight.

My mother had always bemoaned the fact that she hadn't gotten a boob job as a younger woman. "Those were the Marilyn Monroe days," she said, crestfallen. "I was flat as a board and tiny. That wasn't what the boys wanted." (Of course, by the time I was a young woman, her ninety-five-pound frame would have been considered the very height of desirability.) Then she'd brighten. "You should fix your nose, honey. I know it makes you self-conscious."

She wasn't wrong about that. It did. I had a profile that could best be described as "sloping," an overlarge bulb of a nose that cast my mouth and weak chin into shadow. My face looked like the prow of a doleful ship, and I had a lifelong habit of jutting out my chin, trying to counteract the effects, which only made me look like a mutinous bulldog. But I was a feminist; I was against plastic surgery. Wasn't I?

Maybe not. A beautiful friend, one of those I quietly thought must be secretly waiting to punk me because surely no one who looked like that *actually* wanted to be friends with me, told the story over drinks one night of her adolescent abduction. "No, *really*," she said, hands on her temples, eyes wide. "It was like the ten o'clock news gone wrong. I was walking down my suburban street, and a white van pulled up, and a man jumped out of the passenger seat and got his arm around my neck and wrestled me into the back."

We were all agog, wineglasses uncharacteristically forgotten at our elbows. "Holy shit! What did you *do*?"

"Nothing. I mean, I kicked and tried to yell, but I could barely breathe. A neighbor was looking out the window and called the cops, and they came before the van could drive away. But not before they smashed the shit out of my nose trying to get me through the door."

I considered her perfect profile. "But it looks fine now."

She spread her hands on each side of her face and wiggled her fingers: fairy dust. "Dr. Magic Hands. He fixed everything up."

A problem to solve, rather than vanity to appease: that kind of framing was just the excuse I was looking for.

A week later, I was in Dr. Magic Hands's office for a consultation. He took photos of my face from all angles and projected them on the wall, all my faults in stark relief. "So you don't want to do anything too drastic with the nose," he said thoughtfully. I opened my mouth to protest—Why was I doing this, if I wasn't going to be transformed into a ravishing beauty?—and he held out a placating hand as he pointed, slicing his hand down the soft slope of my projected face. "I'd just take this top line down a bit. The real change will be in your chin. We can bolt in a piece of silicone right here"—he pointed to each side of my face—"and it will make your whole face stronger."

Strong: that sounded good, even if I couldn't get the image of Frankenstein's monster and his neck bolts out of my head. A few weeks later, I found myself in what looked like a dentist's chair, a sweet-faced anesthesiologist putting a needle in my arm. I woke up with a face so puffy it could have lifted into the sky, and I slept for a full day on my triumphant mother's couch.

A few days later, I pulled the gauze dressing out of my sinuses, and it was like a magician pulling an endless chain of bright knotted handkerchiefs out of her mouth; I hadn't realized that your sinuses are basically the entire interior of your skull. My eyes were bloodshot and my undereyes bruised. A woman in the supermarket looked at me horrified and whispered, "Honey, you can leave him. You really can," and scuttled away. Gorgeous Friend brought over ice cream, crap magazines, and frothy DVDs, and we watched from the comfort of my futon while I awaited my Beauty Unveiling.

It wasn't a dramatic difference. I started going out again once the swelling hit the size of my original nose, and it receded over such a long time that no one else noticed. But I noticed. My new face marked a mental line in the sand: Before and After. For the first time in my life, I felt attractive. I felt like I belonged. I no longer walked into rooms and immediately felt like a burden to everyone in them. I no longer skulked around the edges of parties, or ducked my head when talking. I wore better-fitting clothing. Almost immediately, I interviewed for, and got, a new, better-paying job.

And a few weeks after pulling those miles of gauze out of my nose, I met Laura.

CHAPTER 7

Breaking It Off

We were introduced at a day-after-Thanksgiving party, thirty people crammed into a teeny apartment, thrilled to be away from the tumult of their families. I had hosted the holiday at my mother's, partly so she wouldn't be alone and partly because she had a dining table. She'd pounded it for attention as we were passing the pie around, stilling the conversation of the friends I'd brought over. She was wearing a pink gingham shirt and every piece of costume jewelry she owned simultaneously; her chest clanked with necklaces. "Girls!" she cried, Queens accent broad with her single glass of red wine. "*Girls*." When she had our attention, she pointed around the table, peering over her bifocals. "It's Thanksgiving. It's a day for thinking about what's important in life. So I'm going to tell you what's important. First," and she raised a finger, "God." Indulgent smiles from the crowd, most of whom were devout atheists. "Second: family." More smiles followed, and nods. "Third: money." The smiles faltered. "And fourth," and here she gestured grandly at her plumage, "BLING."

She had started taking a lot of tranquilizers to manage strangers. It showed.

So I was, needless to say, hungover the next day. I had noticed Laura, floppy haired and tight T-shirted, across the party; she was clutching a plastic cup of water and looking mildly panicked and out of place. The hostess introduced us, beaming; we leaned in shyly and talked. I told her about my work as a science fiction editor, she told me about her days in culinary school. We stood close together, gesturing with our cups and laughing nervously. I gave her my card. She called to offer to make me dinner. I took the N train all the way from Queens through Manhattan into Brooklyn, rattling an hour over the tracks, and ate six courses. Well, four. After the second perfectly cooked, beautifully plated main course, we retired to the couch to watch a comedy show, and, my heart thundering in my chest, I kissed her.

A week and a half later, on our third date, she told me she loved me. A few months later she moved in, temporarily, while she looked for a condo to buy. It was a terrible cliché, but we were happy. Of course I loved living with a chef—who wouldn't?—and my tiny kitchen soon overflowed with branches of unfamiliar dried peppers, a dozen kinds of vinegar, clumps of Buddha's hand, and containers of homemade ice cream. We lived together with my grumpy, middle-aged tuxedo cat, Elvis, in the studio apartment I'd moved into when my roommate Alexa bought her own place, and barely moved from bed except to hit the refrigerator. With not much more than three-hundred square feet to rattle around in, it's a good thing it was the *beginning* of our relationship.

I had never met anyone like Laura before. Raised in Virginia and educated at a fancy, expensive boarding school in New England, she was the child of an acrimonious divorce between a Northeastern Jewish father and the daughter of southern Evangelicals. She was close to her mother, troublingly so, I thought, although I knew I was far from unbiased about what a healthy mother-daughter relationship should look like. And so I kept my mouth shut when her mother's merest disapproving grimace made her cry, when she moved heaven and earth—and our vacation plans—to accommodate her visits, when it became achingly clear that I would never be the first woman in her life. "Therefore shall a man leave his mother and his father, and cleave unto his wife" is very good advice, but Laura never un-cleaved from her mother, who remained her first call with good news and bad. I should have known that this was a bad sign, but I didn't. I thought that maybe this was what a good relationship with your mom looked like. Maybe this was the natural opposite of cringing when you saw your mother's name on the caller ID.

There was a class element to my bewilderment, too. Like my first girlfriend, Caroline, she was just . . . fancier than I was. I was horrified that she remained on her mother's cell phone plan, along with her sister. "But she can see your *records*, she can see who you *called*," I argued, frustrated that I couldn't say what I wanted to: You're an adult, how are you OK with your mother paying your bills, where's your pride? "But it costs less for everyone," she said reasonably. "Why would we pay the phone company more?"

Why! I would have paid them whatever they asked to codify my independence from my mother. Laura thought I was nuts.

We moved into that condo, which Laura and her mother owned jointly, and lived together for five years, reasonably happy. We both loved to travel and took off for big trips every few years—Portugal, New Zealand, China—and we threw brunch and dinner parties where she cooked, performing pan flips and knife skills that made all the guests gasp and cheer. We went to a lot of parties, most thrown by my friends, where she was exhausted by nine p.m. but refused to go home, blinking and swaying silently while conversations swirled around her, until I finally got our coats. I knew we didn't have much in common—either in worldview or habit—but I was ready for The Relationship, and she was cute and nice and she loved me, and that was enough for twenty-nine-year-old me. (I am not proud of this now, mind you.)

When she took a new job a hundred miles south in Camden, New Jersey, she commuted by Amtrak daily for a few months, but she couldn't stand the six-hour round-trip trek and rented a tiny apartment—a converted hotel room, which she shared with a fleet of roaches the size of cats—in Philadelphia. We ended up buying a two-bedroom condo for her to live in, calculating that a roommate's contribution to the mortgage would offset enough to make it a solid investment. And for three years, she lived on the top floor of a Center City walk-up flooded with light and furnished with her grandmother's cast-offs. She came home on weekends, and I visited when I could. When the alarm system tripped one morning during one of those visits, I found out that although she was the first number on the account, the backup was her mother, six hundred miles away. I glanced at her insurance paperwork, tossed on a table; her mother was her emergency contact, too. Why wasn't it me? I asked, astonished. "She's a *doctor*," said Laura, looking at me as if I'd grown a third head. "She's an *anesthesiologist*," I shot back. "How's that going to help her make good end-of-life decisions for you?" She sighed and shook her head. What did I, with my semi-estrangement from my crazy mother, know about anything?

I didn't feel entitled to say, "You should be casting in your lot with me. I should be the most important." I was afraid to hear the obvious truth: I wasn't.

A large part of me enjoyed living alone during the week, which, in retrospect, should have been an armada's worth of red flags. I loved going to readings and parties and events and getting home at midnight with no one cranky and asleep on my shoulder. I loved making weeknight margaritas with a neighbor and dancing in the living room. I loved not having to check her schedule before making plans with all my friends, even people I knew she didn't like, or didn't like her. I had a sneaking thought, which I was too afraid to put into words, that most of the events I went to were more fun without her; leaving concerts and shows we went to together, I would ask, "What was your favorite song?" and she'd look at me as if I'd asked her to solve a complex equation. We had less to say to each other than I'd hoped, but maybe, I thought, this was what relationships were like, after years together. I'd read all the articles, I'd heard all the podcasts. I knew better than to think my partner should be my everything. But she wasn't feeling like quite enough something, either.

Because what I really wanted—what I was ashamed to admit I needed—was a wife.

I wanted to be married. I loved the idea of facing the world as a team, of forming a family that I had actually chosen, rather than the troubled one into which I'd been born. I wanted that intimacy and partnership. This longing made me feel a little like an archaic throwback. I knew very few married couples, and even fewer queer ones. When marriage equality passed in New York State, I ran out of Shabbat services with the rest of my congregation into the streets of Chelsea, hooting and hollering, pirouetting and hugging strangers. When the *Obergefell* decision came down I exploded out of my office chair, screaming and crying. My colleagues ran into my office, alarmed, saw the headline on my screen, and shouted. One picked me up and spun me around. Another started up a jazzy, off-key rendition of "Here Comes the Bride." Ninety-five percent of me was so thrilled to see progress in a country that felt every day like it was moving further toward Christian sharia law and sliding backward. The other five percent was mourning, because I knew Laura would never marry me.

She had given all the truly dumbest reasons, the ones you usually hear from nineteen-year-olds batting new ideas around in dorm rooms in the middle of the night. "It's just a piece of paper." (Surely, surely, a queer person should know better.) "I don't believe in marriage." ("It's not *fairies*," I finally snapped, and she had the good horse sense not to say it again.) When she opened her mouth I heard her mother's voice come out: the mother who still blamed her father for the financial terms of their twenty-five-years-old divorce, and who strongly hinted to both her daughters that only parental love was really real, really forever, and romantic love an inevitable disappointment. Out for dinner right after *Obergefell*, friends asked excitedly if we were going to get married; "God, no," she said, laughing, and my friends politely changed the subject as my face burned.

I tried not to let it rattle me. We'd be *fine*, I told myself. We were a couple, no matter what. My emotional rope was already taken up by my mother, anyway, who called and screamed and hung up and called back and screamed some more. Rattled by her reluctant outreaches to ask for money—calls that had started coming with increasing frequency soon after I graduated from college—I offered to have her bills simply come to me so that I could pay them directly. She wouldn't have to ask, and I wouldn't have to say yes; I would just pay, and the electricity would stay on. She agreed immediately. Her dependence embarrassed her. Some part of her still thought of herself as that newly minted lawyer, buying an apartment with her own money, outfitting it with all-white furniture and a single pop of color from the crystal candy bowl of M&M's, living independently. She woke up each groundhoggy day to the shock of being broke, alone, and nearly housebound, with no tools at her disposal to make the best of it. And she raged each time at the unfairness of it all. Better just to pay the bills silently, no discussion needed.

Torsten saw her more than I did. We were still friends, years after breaking up—he was now married to a college friend of mine—and he and my mother maintained a (to me) inexplicable friendship, one in which every few months he would let her lean on his arm all the way down to the neighborhood diner, where they argued at top volume about politics and she criticized his food choices—bacon and white bread and plain burgers. "You're such a *WASP*," she'd spit out as his order arrived, giving the word the four letters she felt it deserved. He just shook his head and chuckled at her. They got along gangbusters and I was thrilled that she had someone to bring her a sliver of the outside world. Someone who wasn't me.

During her depressive periods, she called me regularly with

a list of instructions for her funeral. She had never planned to live this long. Her mother had died so young, and she'd expected to be long gone already. Why hadn't God taken her yet? she raged, and prayed nightly to be swiftly dispatched in her sleep. During one year she called so often—once a week or so—that I kept the list on my phone so I could repeat it back to her to speed the process up. Traditional shroud, check. Old Montefiore Cemetery next to her mother, check. Only the graveside prayers, check. No eulogy, check. I once blithely related this list in the back of a cab with the president of the synagogue's board, on our way to a meeting. I had forgotten how odd it sounded to strangers until I caught the stunned, sad expression on his face.

One summer afternoon, my phone rang just as the Q train came above ground in Brooklyn. I was on my way back from a weekend in Fire Island with a colleague and her burlesque-dancer girlfriend; Laura had left early to go back to work. I was sunburned and tired and felt, as usual, like a Bad Queer. I lacked so much as an undercut or a visible tattoo, and I was terrible at meeting people at tea dances. It was Mom's phone number, and I steeled myself.

"Hey, Mom."

"Elizabeth?" Her voice was faraway and weak.

I sat up. "Who else calls you Mom? Is everything OK?"

"Not really. I'm sorry. I'm sorry." And she started crying.

"Mom, what on earth? What's going on?"

"This is embarrassing and stupid. So stupid. But I fell, and my legs . . . I can't get back into bed."

"Was this just now?" I racked my brain for the name of her current roommate. "Can Jake help you?"

"No, he left for the weekend on Friday."

Suspicion rose like bile. "Mom, *when did you fall?*"

A moment of silence, and a grunt as she adjusted. "What time is it now? I think about this time yesterday."

"*Yesterday*. You've been on the floor since *yesterday*." The doors opened and I darted off the train, crossing the platform for the one bound back into Manhattan. "OK. I'm coming."

I still had a key. I let myself in and could tell immediately that the air had changed. The apartment usually smelled strongly of cigarette smoke and pungent air freshener, but now I smelled ammonia. Urine.

She was on her back on the floor next to her bed. She'd pulled an afghan down under her head, and had her arms crossed over her then-considerable stomach. She was wearing a pink crepey muumuu, and her hair was matted under her head. She rolled her eyes around in my direction. "Took you long enough to get here," she said crossly. I glared, and she relented. "Oh, Elizabeth, I'm just cranky. I'm all cramped up down here."

I knelt down next to her. "What happened?"

"It's this neurogenic claudication foolishness. My legs get tingly and numb, and if I'm standing up I just go right down." I looked at her legs jutting out from under the housedress, laced with spider veins.

"Can you feel them now?"

She huffed, twitched her toes. "Not a lot."

"OK. I think we need to get you into the bed, first of all, just to get you off the floor. Can you lean up with me?"

A fleeting expression of embarrassment and guilt crossed her face. "Elizabeth, I . . . I shit myself. I couldn't help it." Sure enough, the smell in her room was stronger and earthier than in the hallway.

"It's fine. Let's get you up."

I got behind her and hooked my elbows under her shoulders, pulled upward; no luck. I pushed while she tried to get her elbows onto the bed. I finally squatted, wrapped my arms around her waist, and heaved; she shouted and flopped forward, and we got the top half of her body onto the bed. Holding her shoulders down with one hand, I stepped over her and hoisted her lower half on, my heel squishing in shit. Her eyes squeezed shut and she started crying.

"I didn't put down a pad! The *sheets*!"

She had peed again on touchdown.

Safe in the bed, she shouted directions, and I pawed through the bathroom cabinets for puppy pads and her closet for a clean nightgown. *How long has this been happening that she has puppy pads at the ready*, I kept thinking, but I put the thought from my mind and concentrated on the task at hand. By rolling her back and forth, we got her mopped up and into clean Depends and a clean nightgown. I scrubbed down the floor with bleach and brought her a sandwich. She set it down on her bedside table, her eyelids heavy, and waved me out the door.

I rode back to Brooklyn with a pounding head. I was used to a mother who would call me a hundred times over a dozen weeks, fretting that she might, maybe, someday fall. I didn't know what to make of a mother who would lie for a full day in her own shit before she picked up the phone.

❖ ❖ ❖

Mental illness was now vying with dementia. Her behavior got more and more erratic, and I woke up each day tense, not sure what was going to end up on my voice mail or when I was going to have to drop everything to take the train uptown and get her up off the floor or intervene in a screaming fight with a tenant.

Being raised by a mentally ill parent is like being raised by wolves. Worse than wolves. Holograms, maybe, or an ectoplasmic something that shifts its form, that can look like a normal human being to the people around you but reverts to its monster shape behind closed doors. You didn't go to normal-people school, and so they constantly surprise you. You constantly surprise them, too. You're operating with a different playbook, and just when you think you've got it down, you unknowingly let the zipper on your human suit show. My dearest friend Claire, the most kind and loving woman who has ever lived, once hissed in a quick breath of pain when her toddler son accidentally kicked her in the face while doing a flip. The world went white, and in three seconds I was across the room with him under my arm, having grabbed him away and out of hand's reach. The succession of expressions that crossed her face—confusion, realization, sadness—have stayed with me to this day. Of course she wouldn't have belted him one. But my muscle memory thought she might.

There is no terra firma. Anyone could have done anything; there is no act so terrible as to be beyond the best person you know. That's the most vicious part of telling someone such compelling lies. You teach them that they can be fooled. You show them how shitty their own judgment is. You let them know their own minds can't be trusted.

✦ ✦ ✦

I traveled a lot. By then I was working for a company based in the Midwest, and once a month I packed my things and decamped for a week to a Holiday Inn right off frozen Lake

Michigan. My colleagues didn't know what to make of me and I didn't know what to make of them. They had never met a Jew before; I had never met anyone who'd never met a Jew before. They saw my sarcasm as rudeness, and I saw their pleasantly blank faces as we talked, their lack of interrupting or engaging, the same way. We got used to each other in time, but I always felt like an alien wandering a strange land wearing insufficient snow boots.

Grand Haven is a resort town that swells to bursting during the brief summer weeks and empties out the rest of the year. I spent my nights there drinking in the handful of town bars and arguing about politics in the hotel bar, where I ate most of my dinners. Western Michigan is the Bible Belt of the North, and I didn't get far in those arguments. I had never driven on a regular basis, and I found the temporary familiarity of the rental cars thrilling. On more than one occasion, I crossed the bridge over the dark Grand River during those long winter nights and pictured what would happen if I just kept driving. Past Spring Lake. Past Muskegon. Over the Mackinac Bridge to the Upper Peninsula, and on into Canada, the darkness of the North Pole ahead.

It did not occur to me that happy people generally don't fantasize with quite that much fervor about disappearing.

I knew I was drinking too much. There was nothing else to do in Grand Haven most of the year, and beer helped blunt the edges of my loneliness, both in the artful-shades-of-gray Holiday Inn and on my own couch as Laura and I stared at each other, trying to come up with something to talk about. After a dinner party one night I found myself finishing a departed guest's wine as I cleaned up, Laura long since in bed, and I thought, uneasily: this isn't normal. My mother almost never drank, and working in publishing—a boozily friendly industry—had given me, I started to think, an off-kilter idea of what normal drinking was, and what problem drinking was. I dialed it back, but when things got bad in my own head, beer solved it. I still have a faint scar on one knee from a late-night encounter with a lamppost. The lamppost won.

✦ ✦ ✦

I was never much of a fan of Laura's sister Alana, but she was my family now, and we dutifully packed up and went to visit her in her echoing townhouse in the Boston suburbs twice a year. Eight years in, we went up for her birthday. We had been having a hard summer. Laura was having something like a third-life crisis, edgy and perennially disappointed, bursting into occasional soliloquies about the piano lessons she'd failed to take and the places she'd never been. *We live apart five days of the week, what's stopping you from taking the damn piano lessons*, I thought, but didn't say. She was also getting broody, gazing at babies in restaurants and making mawkish references to the children she'd planned to raise with her mother if she stayed single, the kids she would now never have. Because—unspoken—of me.

So we were quiet and a little awkward as we drove to Boston for Alana's birthday party, a subdued dinner affair where as an afterthought she served a single bottle of wine, a bottle that turned out to be the vinegared dregs left in the bottom of last year's birthday dinner wine. In the middle of the meal, her phone rang and a distraught stranger was on the other side; she'd found texts from Alana's number on her boyfriend's phone. "I didn't know he had a girlfriend," she said, shrugging.

Not her problem, clearly; she had a history of sleeping with married men, and my only surprise was that she hadn't known this one was spoken for, rather than just not caring that he was. Laura spent most of the night in the bathroom, pleading an upset stomach. The friends filed home after a desultory dessert.

The next morning, I was standing at the guest bathroom sink scrubbing my teeth when Laura's work phone, plugged into the only accessible outlet, made a peculiar pinging sound. It wasn't her usual text notification, and it wasn't my own phone, jammed into my pajama pocket.

In a heartbeat, I thought of the closed bathroom door. The times that month that I'd woken up in the middle of the night to find her turned away from me, screen glowing over her shoulder. The weight loss, the tighter pants, the sudden lack of semi-annoyed stories about what "that idiot intern Jamie" had fucked up that week.

I eyed the phone consideringly, toothbrush walrus-ing out of my mouth. I'm a great believer in privacy. I had told her, often, that I could forgive an affair, but that if she ever read my journal, she'd never hear my voice again. Clearly, my bluff was being called.

I picked up the phone. It was unlocked. There was only one app on the second screen, and only one contact in the WhatsApp account, which I'd never known her to use. I clicked it open.

You've seen this rom-com and you know this story. A string of texts—*I kiss you, I kiss you, I kiss you*—more reminiscent of a middle-school crush than they were the artifacts of an adult affair. And yet that's what it was. A week's worth of fervent mush, dating from the ill-fated trip upstate to the remote riverside home of a friend, where she had shooed us all into an ice cream stand on the way home and stayed in the car where she finally had cell service, mysteriously absent for twenty minutes, finally emerging flushed and guilty and pocketing her phone to find us mopping up the sticky table, long done. In the months later, it was that moment that haunted me, the starving urgency that had her bent over her phone before we were all fully out of the car, desperate for a bar of service. She couldn't stand another moment without her.

The cliché isn't just a cliché. My heart was cold. My whole body was cold. My teeth clacked together, my head went blank. I yanked the phones off their cables—later, meanly, I regretted not messaging something pithy and gleeful back to the Other Woman when I had the chance—and charged back into the bedroom. She was turning over in bed.

"Get. The fuck. Up," I bit out.

She knew immediately what had happened, but panicked, fudged. "What's going on?"

I threw her work phone down on the bed. "Get the fuck up, you cheat. Get up. You're driving me home."

She looked down at the phone. I was still holding her personal one. "What did you—"

"You know what I saw. What the fuck, Laura. What the fuck. An *intern*, for fuck's sake. What is wrong with you?"

Her eyes were helpless, cornered, but I also saw relief in there. She had been found out, the grenade she'd thrown had exploded, and now she could finally start packing. My life in shards around me, I snapped, enraged, "Maybe I should ask Jamie what the fuck is wrong with *her*."

For the first time, I saw a glimmer of fear in her face. For the first time, I had said something that got through. She lunged across the bed toward the phone. "No!"

"Aha," I said softly. "Well. Now we know who you care about."

I started throwing my clothes into my suitcase, willy-nilly. Silently, she joined me. She went downstairs as I packed up the bathroom, and I came down to hear her telling Alana what had happened. I set down my bag and hugged her. "It looks like we probably won't see each other again, so thanks for always being so nice to me," I said stupidly. She made a noncommittal noise and averted her eyes. This was my own lie. She'd been perfectly and superficially pleasant to me, but I was peripheral at best in that family. The most welcome thing that would come from this breakup, I already knew—if it was a breakup—was that I would never again have to third-wheel it in this already-complete family unit.

We got in the car and started the long drive south. I don't remember everything that was said during that weepy, screaming, tempestuous ride. I remember buying yogurt and a hard-boiled egg at a rest stop, the only food I thought I could choke down, and coming out to find her quickly hanging up the phone. I remember demanding that she stop speaking to Jamie immediately—I still thought, then, that we were navigating an infidelity, not carrying out the steps of a breakup long choreographed—and was told calmly that she had to speak to her for at least another week, as she was delivering the cake to Jamie's wedding the following weekend.

The cake.

That cake—"That Fucking Cake," as it became known to my friends—became the symbol to which I clung to remind myself that something was insane here, someone had gone totally off the rails, but it wasn't me. You don't leave a long-time partner for a crush and then help cater that crush's wedding. You just don't.

I started laughing and couldn't stop. She shifted her fingers nervously on the wheel. "What?"

"I just. I can't." I laughed, hiccupped, started laughing again. "Do you not understand how badly you've allowed yourself to be used?"

Her hands jerked and her voice was hard. "I don't know what you're talking about."

"Well, let's tally this up, shall we? She gets her piece on the side, she gets to feel irresistible, she gets her fucking wedding cake delivered, and, at the end of the day, she still gets her wife. What do *you* get?"

She was silent. I think until that moment it had not occurred to her that she was using this absurd situation to leave a relationship, or that the Other Woman had an agenda of her own; she was flying high on a romantic fantasy, and while she had seen as far as the car ride to deliver the shining white cake, she had not contemplated the solo car ride home.

When the endless hours had passed and we got home, I slammed into the bathroom to wash my burning, swollen face. I heard the bed creak under her weight, and her soft voice greet her mother's call. "No," she said. "No. I'm not in Philadelphia yet. I drove Liz back to Brooklyn."

And I heard Joan's voice, sharp through the phone line: "Well. That wasn't exactly convenient for you. How long will it take you to get home?"

Later, when I remembered her mother's sniping about relationships and marriage, her constant snide comments about the futility of love, and the visible advantage of having two single—or effectively single—daughters who would drop everything to be with her, I also remembered that phone call. To hear your daughter confess that she had cheated, that she had hurt someone, that she had thrown a hand grenade into her relationship, and to find all this so unremarkable—so inevitable, even—that your only comment is on the momentary inconvenience presented by a long drive, this threw the dysfunction of that relationship into stark relief. Joan cultivated immaturity in Laura, I suspected, because it turned her into a lifelong child, and gave Joan someone to mother anew and again. She didn't want to marry again, she'd told us, but she treated her daughters like her primary family, her home team, and they obliged. Laura had never really had space in her life for a partner. And here we were.

To make matters even more exciting, Joan and a friend were staying with "us" that weekend. They were out sightseeing. When the door clicked shut behind Laura, I took the cats and their accoutrements, a bottle of scotch and a glass, and a jar of peanuts into the bedroom and shut the door behind me. I tunneled into the closet and wedged myself under a hanging rack. And I picked up my phone and started dialing. What the *fuck*, I said to each friend in turn. Not one of them could tell me.

The next morning, I was up at five. I showered and dressed as quietly as I could, eased the bedroom door open, and tiptoed down the hall and through the living room. The cats shot past me, yowling. I shut the apartment door behind me and breathed a sigh of relief. And then I looked down at my feet. Slippers.

I stomped and cursed softly. I wiggled the key into the lock and opened the door again, and came face to face with Joan, who stood frozen in the doorway, a mug and a box of herbal tea in her hands. "Forgot my shoes," I said dumbly. She stood back, and I retrieved them. *Don't leave like this*, I thought. *You're an adult.* "Joan, thank you for always being so nice to me," I replayed. "I don't think we'll see each other again after today." Her mouth dropped open and her eyes—Were those *tears*? What on *earth*? "Oh honey, *no*!" She gasped. "Don't say that!" She hugged me, fiercely. I said something vague and scrambled out the door, safely shod. I never spoke to her again.

The next weeks were a blur. I choked down oatmeal in the mornings and shunned food the rest of the day, dropping ten pounds in as many days. Claire called twice a day from Michigan, making sure I hadn't fallen off the edge of the earth, and listened, baffled, to my questions that no one could answer: What happened? Why now? What did she want? Why the *intern*, for the love of all that was holy? Who picked such a maudlin, embarrassing cliché on which to turn one's life? Claire and I had had the kind of friendship you see in buddy movies, where since college we had talked nearly every day about everything and nothing. Now she listened helplessly to me weeping, unable to come up with a plausible explanation.

My mother called, and I debated just failing to mention what had happened, but it came rushing out, my voice breaking. She broke in: "Oh Elizabeth, *no*. I'm so sorry. You have to meet someone else! It is so terrible to be alone. Loneliness is the worst thing in the world!" I knew she was talking about herself. I still ended the call with a vicious poke to the screen, wishing I had a handset to slam down.

Guylaine, to whom I'd stayed close since our breakup and who was in New York on a spur-of-the-moment road trip, met me for smoothies on a park bench and listened to my story silently, holding my hands in hers. "This sadness is not forever. Someday it will be over, and you will be better," she said.

"But how do you *know*," I wailed.

"There's something we say in French," she said, a small smile quirking her lips. "Can I tell you?"

I wiped my eyes and chuckled. "Yeah, OK, hit me with your Francophone wisdom."

She spread her hands, then dropped them sharply into her lap. "Ça passe, ou ça casse," she said simply. "It passes, or it breaks."

Laura and I had planned to take two weeks apart to consider the situation, and what we wanted—to part so that we would stop clawing at each other. I had a planned trip to visit my college friend Caitlin in Syracuse en route to a work trip, and for the full weekend we hiked, we ate ice cream, and we drank strong gin and tonics on her porch, brought to us by her soft-spoken professorial husband, who paused on his way inside after delivering fresh glasses to say cautiously: "I don't want to intrude, Liz. But this is some bullshit."

It was.

There was traffic on the way back to the Syracuse airport, and I was running late, and the TSA agents behaved as all TSA agents in small airports do; they went through every inch of my carry-on twice, and when I fidgeted, they slowed down. I made it onto the plane by the skin of my teeth and it wasn't until we were midair and I was peering down the aisle for the drinks cart that I realized that my laptop was still in the airport scanner.

My small company was a subsidiary of Amazon, giving it the worst possible mix of Midwestern passive-aggression and tech-giant stress. Their security requirements were draconian, and I knew before I asked that even if the airport would agree to ship the laptop to me in Michigan, Amazon policy did not allow laptops to be mailed. I bumbled through a week in the office with a loaner laptop, eating too little and lying rigid in the hotel bed each night, staring at the ceiling, my stomach roiling. I went out to drinks with the studio head, who said hesitantly, "You look like you haven't been eating," and I put my head down on the bar and sobbed.

At six a.m. on the last morning of my trip, without any better ideas in mind, I canceled my return flight, and started driving.

I couldn't go the most direct route because it ran across a spike of Canada and of course I didn't have my passport. So I drove down and around, all the way across Michigan, all the way across Ohio, all the way across Pennsylvania, watching hundreds of miles of farmland unspool along the heat-shimmering highway. I remember feeling a rush of gratitude—an emotion that had been in short supply—that it was August and not the dead of winter, when the lake effect turned the western shore of Michigan into a single dark-laned ice slick, and when it snowed so hard that I would get off the highway if I couldn't find a truck to follow, its giant brake lights a guide through the whiteout.

It was summer. The trees shifted and rustled above me, and at a gas station where I stopped for more Coke Zero and sour gummy worms, a little girl in a bathing suit, still wet from a sprinkler, ran past me yelling a song from *Frozen*. This vast country—a quarter of which I was driving across in a single day—was full of people who were happy, who were vacationing, who didn't know that the woman I loved had spent the weekend delivering a wedding cake to the woman she, in turn, loved.

In fairness, had they known, they wouldn't have believed me. That Fucking Cake! That Fucking Cake.

In Syracuse, I followed the GPS into the office park of buildings that supported the airport. A receptionist took my name, and did I imagine that her eyes widened slightly? "Oh yes," she said, "you're the one who called. One minute." And she disappeared, stepping quickly. Had I been crying when I called them? I couldn't remember. It was a safe bet.

Laptop once again safely in my hands—it took all my meager self-possession not to spike that troublesome fucker at the floor—I turned south and headed back to the city, leaving the rental car at LaGuardia Airport in the middle of a rainstorm that flooded out the sidewalks and blurred the lights. I had driven 950 miles in sixteen straight hours. I crawled into bed still dressed and slept, blessedly dream-lessly, until the alarm shrilled me awake for work.

A few days later, right before the planned meeting and the end of those enervated, acid-stomached two weeks, Laura reached out cheerfully over GChat to let me know she'd be back that weekend and how excited she was for a haircut; she then broke up our relationship of eight years over instant message. Looking back, I can only laugh. She had been out of that rela-tionship since long before the Car Ride of Doom. She was dizzy with the new vista that had opened before her. She was flying to the sun. I had been reeling from shock and trying to catch up, but it was now clear: she had been gone for a long time.

I closed my laptop and sat on my hands, trying to keep them from shaking. The apartment was silent, the noisy bus stop below the living room windows momentarily unoccupied and still.

I got my phone and started texting. I have never been someone who wants to work through things alone; I crowd-source everything and rely on others for a gauge of sanity.

Claire, who had called twice a day to make sure I was making it through; Caitlin, at whose home I spent the weekend after the Car Ride of Doom; and Kat, the friend whose ex-partner had turned out, two years into living together, to have been carrying on a turbulent and engrossing affair the entire time. ("Laura turned out to be Emily," I texted her succinctly as I waited for Laura to pack up the car at Alana's, and she understood immediately.) Kat got back to me first. "I'm at the Austin airport waiting to get on a flight," she responded. "Are you home? I can be there in six hours."

Six hours later, the doorbell rang and there she was, a functional person fresh from the real world, with her carry-on backpack filled to bursting with beer and chips from the bodega downstairs. I took one of the wine bottles Laura the Teetotaler had brought back from a work trip to Paris—the only act of destruction or revenge that I took, which I'm still pretty fucking proud of—and squeaked it open. We sat at the kitchen island and drank it, and we talked, and I cried. She had survived a worse, more calculated betrayal, a phone full of texts of sweet nothings identical to the words just said to her, a long bathroom visit during a restaurant dinner after which a strangely familiar young woman traipsed past their table and out the door, smugly flushed and rumpled. She knew what it was to wake up in Wonderland, to find that the world in which you had just woken up was not the world in which you went to sleep, and never was. This was a premeditated lie, a lie that was told for the thrill of putting one over on someone. And Kat had survived. Beautiful, brilliant Kat. If she could, I could.

Eventually.

If I could never know what was true, I decided, I was just going to go for the gold. I would enjoy the shit out of myself.

People lied. This was a fact like gravity or seasons. You could never, ever know for sure if what was being said to you was true. The trick was not to care. If you don't care, it won't matter.

I still wept myself to sleep at night and awake in the morning. But in between, I steeled myself. Back in the world, I instructed myself firmly. Back on the horse.

The next few weeks looked like a movie montage of a recent breakup, preferably with myself played by Kristen Wiig. I had been in a nearly sexless relationship for the better part of a decade, and I was ready to splash out. With nothing to lose, I got brazen. A good-looking friend of a friend reached out with condolences, and after ten minutes of semi-flirtatious Facebook messaging—he was known for being an outrageous flirt and, armed with a charming accent and a career in female-heavy publishing, a successful one—I had propositioned him and his wife, both of whom I immediately started dating. "Dating," of course, being defined as whiskey-fueled nights tumbling laughing into generic Midtown hotel rooms, clutching champagne bottles by the neck, and cheerfully tossing underwear onto lampshades. We all needed to feel beautiful and exciting, and this was the moment. I loved the proximity to their happy, sexy relationship, a reminder that there were such things in the world.

I also called Arie.

CHAPTER 8

Switching Teams

We'd fallen out of touch every now and then, but Arie and I had stayed friends through high school, college, our ridiculous twenties and responsible thirties. He took leave from his fancy law-firm job to do volunteer legal work in Cambodia and Uganda. Every winter he took all his vacation time in one month, scuba diving in various remote locations and coming home with a beard that made him look like a conflict zone photographer. I joked that it was like being friends with James Bond. He dated some of my friends; I tagged along on some of his crazier endeavors. He was always the first to know about some weird new site-specific theater event, an all-night Robyn dance party, a citywide scavenger hunt or pillow fight.

We had some history between us, more sexual than romantic. At fifteen, we kissed on my mother's kitchen floor during a group sleepover, he trembling like a linden; at nineteen, he drove from Staten Island with his newly acquired license to visit me in my dorm room; at twenty-six, my girlfriend and I were looking for someone to have a threesome with, and I thought about who I knew who was sexy, fun, and wouldn't be an asshole about the offer, and he came up cherries on all fronts. So we had, you know, a bit of *history*. We'd always had a spark, but he also always had girlfriends. As had I.

He and Laura got along like a house on fire. He was always on board for her ambitious creative projects, and the two of them would render beef fat into soap and roll chocolate truffles while I sat at the counter, drinking wine and laughing with them. Every summer, we biked down to Clemente's in Sheepshead Bay and demolished buckets of all-you-can-eat crabs in rickety plastic chairs overlooking the marina, and then biked home in the twilight stinking to the skies of Old Bay. He came to our parties and laughed at our jokes. When I texted him to say that Laura had left me, and what the *fuck*, he was as baffled as I was.

Did I want to talk? Come on over.

I showed up on his doorstep in the shortest dress I had. He gallantly averted his eyes and installed me on the couch while he ordered dinner. I still wasn't eating, so I got a side serving of sweet potato and forked it desultorily. After dinner we moved to chairs on his giant Brooklyn Heights roof deck overlooking the Manhattan skyline and sat together in silence, breathing, listening to the swish of traffic on the streets below. The August air hung close and heavy, and the city shone bright.

I made my move, awkwardly. "So hey, listen. I have a question for you. And totally fine if the answer is no, no hard feelings." He smiled and opened his mouth to respond, and I rushed ahead: "But I've been having bad, infrequent sex for years, and I'd like to have some great sex, and I'd love it to be with you."

His mouth stayed open for a long moment. He snapped it shut, ducked his head, swallowed, smiled. "I'm flattered. But this doesn't seem like the right time. You're clearly feeling pretty vulnerable right now and I don't want to take advantage of that. And if the two of you get back together, I don't want to have caused trouble in the middle."

"How about you let me worry about that?"

"I can't. But believe me, that is a very flattering offer."

The next week, after Laura broke us off for good, I showed up on his doorstep in tight jeans and a low-cut top. Whatever objections he had left, he managed them on his own.

Ours was not a romance of innocents. For a while, it wasn't a romance at all—just a friendship that suddenly included some really great sex. We had both been in relationships that flared and went wrong, that went right for a long time and then collapsed. We had been on a hundred weird dates and a hundred dull ones. We had known each other since we were bone skinny (him) and acne spattered (me). He put up with me during my hard-party years, and I put up with him during his law school years, when every conversation became an opportunity to argue a case. In twenty-five years, we had never run out of things to talk about. It turns out that spending a lot of time naked with someone only adds to the possible topics.

Slowly, I started eating real food again. We walked for miles after work, stopping for ice cream wherever we could find it. We went out for meals in Brooklyn Heights, walking back hand in hand on the Promenade, looking out over the river. We didn't tell our friends, although of course they knew. On group outings we would arrive separately and leave separately, meeting up around the corner and falling laughing into each other's arms; one night he swung me around and pulled me into a hug in his giant wool overcoat. "Oh *Scheier*," he said gruffly. And I knew, then, that he was falling in love with me, and that I had already been in love with him for a long time.

We ate tacos. We went to the symphony. We went to San Diego for Kat's fortieth birthday, and he sat in a hot tub with a mob of my bikinied friends and kept his eyes steadfastly at eye level. We took a trip to Myanmar, and held each other close in a freezing train bunk overnight from Yangon to Bagan, our friend Alexa politely pretending to sleep above us. We ate durian at a hawker stall in Singapore, hands sheathed in latex gloves to keep off the famous almond-gasoline stench. We dove down to the wreck of the USAT *Liberty* in Bali, where a free diver in a blue-skirted bathing suit kicked sinuously past me toward the far-off sunlit surface, bright bubbles dappling over her body.

In October, I got a call I had long since stopped expecting. The previous year, an old friend, Ed—the director of the summer camp at which Arie and I had met—had posted on Facebook that he needed a kidney, had been on the list too many years, and was losing faith. I messaged him immediately. *I've got two*, I wrote, *you've got zero, let's even this out.*

It's not quite that easy. I went through the two full days of testing, scans and exams and nineteen (yes) vials of blood on a fasting stomach, and a psych evaluation to make sure I could handle it if the transplant wasn't successful. And I was cleared to donate. But like only four percent of the population, my blood type is AB positive. We weren't a match. And before we could find another donor-recipient pair to swap with, he had a heart attack and a bypass. No more surgeries, not for the time being. And so I had checked the box to put myself on the national registry, not wanting to waste all that testing, and more or less forgot about it.

Until now.

When the living donor coordinator called, I was packing to move out of Laura's apartment. I answered the phone from a maze of boxes containing the last eight years of my life, possibly including the cats, whom I hadn't seen since breakfast. She was polite, but urgent. The recipient was twenty-five years old and would be transplanted at Johns Hopkins in Baltimore. Could I come in on Monday for follow-up testing to be sure I was still healthy? Could I have the surgery in two weeks?

I could. I would. I would have washed my dusty face and come in right that moment if they would have let me. I was filled with a freezing wash of exhilaration and relief. Finally, a break from the three months of post-breakup heartache and upheaval. Finally, a question that was easy to answer, unlike the rhetorical paces I'd been putting myself through for months: Why had all this happened? What did I do wrong? What were the chances that I would find love again? It felt fantastic to say an unequivocal, unconcerned *yes*. It felt fantastic to be sure I knew what the right thing was. The miracle of this surgery—an organ that could be unplugged from one person and plugged into another, and *both of them live*—felt like a reprieve, a One Good Thing that could never be taken away.

I was not, as you may remember, planning on having children. There was no sense in saving my extraneous organ. And there was no use in hoarding it in my own body if someone else needed it. Non-relative living transplants can last up to fifteen years. By that time, who knows? We might have synthetic kidneys. We might be able to transplant animal ones. We just had to keep the patients around and alive until then.

My one worry was Ed. He was still waiting for his kidney. If he switched his care to a hospital that participated in the National Kidney Registry, *and* went through all the testing again, *and* was cleared for surgery, *and* if we could find a donor pair to swap with, I could still get him his kidney. Having a willing donor is currency and he had, after all, been the one to bring me into the system. Could I really leave him behind? On the other hand, could I disappoint the anonymous recipient currently counting down the days for surgery against the future possibility of finding someone with AB-positive blood, matching antibodies, a wonky kidney, and a mismatched donor?

I consulted friends, none of whom knew what to tell me. I've rarely run into a moral quandary where I didn't really know perfectly well what the ethical course of action was, and where the challenge wasn't just doing the hard-but-right thing. I had no idea what to do. They didn't either. In a panic, I called my rabbi, and laid it out for her. She didn't skip a beat.

"Are you familiar with the concept of *pikuach nefesh*?" she asked.

". . . Sort of," I said cautiously. "That's the one where you can break any of the Shabbat rules in order to save a life?"

"Correct!" she said. "But we take it a step further. Jewish law values life above all else, and it's more of an active command-ment than a passive one. If you *can* save a life, you *must*. You *may not stand aside* when a life is in danger. In this situation, where it's not clear which life to save, you are in the right whichever path you choose. But, Liz: practicality also plays a part here. You have the opportunity in front of you. Don't set it aside against the possibility that another may—or may not!—arise in the future." *Don't be a nitwit*, I translated silently.

Arie wanted to go with me for the surgery. Absolutely not,

I said. It would be hours before anything interesting happened, and why should he miss work just to sit cooling his heels in a waiting room? I took the subway to the hospital for a six a.m. pre-surgical check-in. The train was silent. I patted the left side of my back and wished Left Kidney a fond farewell. By that time the next morning I would be forever linked to a stranger by a separated set of organs. I thought of those friendship pendants so popular when I was a kid, each comprising a jagged half of a heart, and laughed, nervousness flushing cold through my veins. Godspeed, little kidney. No dying in transit. Show up with your shield or on it.

It all happened so fast that I didn't have time to get frightened until I was on the table, the anesthesiologist's kindly face hovering above my own. I breathed, I counted backward, I woke up in recovery with a Band-Aid over my belly button and a head full of tumbleweeds. A hospital volunteer, a friend from synagogue who'd gotten herself assigned to the recovery room that day, was standing at the foot of the bed with Arie. "He charmed me into letting him in before you were awake," she said, and winked.

I spent only a single night in the hospital, with Arie wedged uncomfortably on a cot next to my bed, wearing an extra hospital gown as pajamas. I was sent home with a bottle of Percocet and, more healing still, a text from the transplant coordinator: "Surgery successful. Kidney adjusting beautifully. Patient will live."

If you have to be in the hospital, take a lawyer with you. Arie sweet-talked the doctor on call into discharging me early and helped me carefully into a cab, settling me into bed with a painkiller and a bag of ice. He stayed with me that whole first day when the pain of the surgical gas was worst, bringing me ice cream and finding me shows on Netflix.

In the long-red-blaze-of-pain days between the Car Ride of Doom and the GChat Breakup, I had written down a list of things I wanted in a partner. I hoped that the list would be definitive one way or another; that it would prove that Laura and I had never been a good match and that I now had a solid path forward, or that we had been a perfect match, and that I should move heaven and earth to convince her that I was a better bet than the Intern Bride. The list was inconclusive but leaned toward the wrong match. Laura had most of the characteristics I wanted in a partner by number, but not by weight. She didn't want to marry me, and I didn't want to raise the children for whom she was pining. Some of our most core values were misaligned. And most importantly, we didn't have good banter. We were totally lacking on the witty repartee score. When I texted her what I thought were pretty good jokes, she texted back "LOL." When I sent her articles I thought were interesting, she never responded. Arie and I had been talking for twenty-five years, and neither of us had gotten bored yet.

He was good, and kind, and brilliant, and hilarious. He was interested in everything and interesting himself as a result. He was a man, it's true, and I hadn't dated one of those since Tor and I had broken up. But from my vantage point curled up in the corner of my couch trying not to move any of my core muscles, I knew: I could see in him the things that I wanted for myself and my future.

I recovered from the surgery. We spent multiple nights a week together. We could no longer deny that what we had was getting serious. Which suited both of us just fine.

But all the time we had this difference between us: he wanted children, and I didn't.

That's not the kind of decision you can compromise on. It's not a choice about where to live, where I want a farm and you want a city so we settle on the suburbs; it's not you finishing your dissertation before I start my master's. There's no middle ground on procreation.

I couldn't even picture how having kids . . . *worked*. My day started at six a.m. when I left for the gym, and ended between ten p.m. and midnight when I got home from whatever I was doing that night. I was on the board of my synagogue, which meant meetings and more meetings; I volunteered one night a week and went to services another. I was involved in half a dozen professional and literary organizations. I went out with friends most other nights. There were maybe three or four days in the whole year when I went straight home from work. This wasn't a life that could easily fit a child, not without a reshaping that took out so many of the things I loved.

And more importantly, I didn't like children. It wasn't a philosophical or aesthetic distaste; *oh get* over *it*, I thought when friends waxed pompously on about the terribleness of diapers and sticky fingers and what have you. I just didn't find them interesting.

"Kids *aren't* interesting," a friend told me bluntly over margaritas when I laid my dilemma out before her. "I can't stand my friends' kids. Or my son's friends. They're all awful. He's the only one I like. It's biology; you've gotta love your own kids or you'd leave them on a hillside like the Spartans to die of exposure."

"That seems like kind of a risk," I said. "What if you *don't*? Now you've ruined your life *and* you're ruining a kid's."

She put down her glass and examined me closely. "You think you're special?"

Should I be insulted? "I mean. Sure I do. Doesn't everyone?"

"You're not smarter than anyone else, sweetheart. Or any different. You'll have them, you'll love them. It'll be a shit-show but it'll be *great*. Give it a shot, why the fuck not?" She downed her drink. "You won't be any worse of a parent than the rest of us."

Strangely, that argument—*you aren't special*—was the one that swayed me. I wasn't any better than anyone else. Nor was I any worse. The odds that I would turn out to be a mother like my own had to be slim; I was no Platonic ideal of emotional perfection, but I wasn't carrying the diagnosis and the history that she had. Maybe this was just a new chapter. I had wanted a certain kind of life, and I'd gotten it. For a long time. I'd had the child-free home, just me and my equally footloose-and-fancy-free partner, and I had been happy. Until I wasn't.

I could try to re-create that, except with someone better suited to me. I could spend the rest of my life looking. Or I could try something else.

Arie was what I wanted. This sweet, funny, endlessly entertained and entertaining person who was congenitally incapable of lying to me. And while he loved his parents, I knew without asking that hell had a greater chance of exploding into ice than he had of listing them as his In Case of Emergency contact rather than his partner. The price of admission to being with him was having kids. If we did, and if the thing I didn't even want to consider happened—if I became my mother and became a danger—he would be there to stop me and save them.

I finally said: Fuck it. Don't wear that condom tonight. And he didn't.

A month later, he woke me up at midnight on Valentine's Day. He was wearing a dapper suit, and had scattered a hundred tulips, my favorite flower, on the floor. He had a speech and he had a ring. His hands shook as he held mine, and when he asked, I was overcome. "Come here," I said gruffly and tried to pull him in for a kiss. "But wait hold on is that a yes," he said, panicked, and yes. It was a yes.

We got dressed—he in his tux, me in the going-out dress he had told me to bring for a Valentine's Day surprise, the closest he could get to a lie—and we stood on the patio in the February midnight and toasted with champagne. He was characteristically tipsy after a few sips. I held his warm hand on the freezing patio and marveled that just six months before, I had wailed in his arms that no one would ever love me again. It was like someone had looked at my life—the breakup, the raging mother, the surgery, the move—and had decided that enough was enough. With all the certainties in my life stripped away, I could see what I had never needed and what I had always wanted. And here he was.

The next morning, we texted friends and called our parents. His parents were thrilled, though probably a little confused—they hadn't heard my name in decades, after all—and my mother pretty much lost her shit. When I told her I was getting married, she screamed in delight, and then said: "Are you pregnant????" I was too happy to yell at her. I met my godparents for our regular monthly dinner and did the cinematic ring flash when I told them; my godmother, Shannon, burst into tears and ran around the booth to hug me. As the burgers arrived, I said, "So you guys have been happily married forever, what's your secret? What's the key to a good marriage?" And simultaneously, Joe said, "Unconditional love," and Shannon said, "Separate vacations."

In retrospect, I think they were both right.

My friends were cautiously thrilled. A lot of them asked, in not as many words, if I was *sure*; it was a big change, after all, and it had been less than six months since Laura swanned out the door. And . . . you know. A man. What was I thinking? they wanted to know. Was I sure?

I was sure. The best part about getting out of a bad relationship is that the bad parts are thrown into such stark relief. The moment your head begins to clear, you think: What? Why did I put up with that? Why did I allow that to happen? Why did I throw away so many years on something that I knew, in the gritty ocean floor of my soul, wasn't right? Why did I ignore the fact that when I'd met Laura, she was carrying on a torrid affair with (yet another) engaged woman? Why, when she slipped and mentioned her active OKCupid account four years in, did I accept her explanation that it was "to find friends" and let her make me feel bad that I'd cut off a potential social connection by demanding she take down her profile? Why did I let my desire to be in a relationship blind me to such blisteringly obvious lies? Why was I so dumb?

Why are any of us so fucking dumb about love, when it's all we want?

Well. No more. Arie was the best person I knew, and I was in love with him. My luck was turning around. I was going to hold on with octopus arms and never let go.

We went to a fertility doctor right away, not because we had any reason to think we'd have trouble but because we were in our late thirties and I wanted to get any fixable problems fixed before we lost any more time. I had an undignified amount of blood drawn. Arie had a specimen cup and a sheepish expression. Everything went off to the lab and I put baby-making out of my mind, hopping the Q train down to Coney Island with a friend visiting from New Zealand. She went to the bathroom at Nathan's and I arranged our chili fries and thirty-two-ounce wax cups of Coors Light on a picnic table, zipping my jacket against the ocean wind. My phone rang; it was the nurse with the results of my blood test. "Hello!" I said cheerfully. "What's the verdict? Find anything terrible?"

"Well, I hope you won't think so!" she said. "The doctor says he's disappointed he can't claim to be responsible for this, but you were already pregnant when you came in."

"Sorry, I . . . say that again?"

"You're about four weeks pregnant," she said, laughing. "Come in again this week so we can make sure your progesterone's up to speed, but congratulations!"

Kim was coming out of the bathroom. I had taken a single sip of my beer, and I pushed it away so hard it sloshed. "Don't *waste*!" she said teasingly.

"You'd better take that," I said grimly, and lied. "That was the kidney follow-up people. They need a clean pee test tomorrow."

"Ha! Sucker." She cheerfully hoisted the beer in her free hand and drank. My head filled with static. *Pregnant.* I had never given any thought to how it might feel. I was completely unprepared.

I drifted around in a daze. I knotted my shirt under my breasts and turned in front of the mirror, hands on hips: still flat. I'd been fired from my job a few months before—sitting under your desk crying after a breakup does not endear you to your boss, it turns out—and had nothing to occupy me except the bizarre, surreal knowledge that there was someone else living in my body. A tiny clump of cells who could one day become someone who hated me as I had, at times, hated my mother. A person I could fuck up to the nth degree without meaning to. A person I had absolutely zero idea how to parent. What had I done?

Arie was thrilled to bits. This was, after all, the man who took the New York State bar exam with barely any prep, and who dove meters beneath the water to catch a glimpse of the fish that wouldn't come see him at the top. In Arie-land, if you want it, you do it, and if you do it, you succeed. We were going to be the best parents. He was sure.

CHAPTER 9

Father Figure

Arie had been offered his dream job with the Department of Justice, and we were looking down the barrel of a move to DC, where we knew almost no one. The FBI was taking its sweet time on his background check and we were cooling our heels, knowing that the moment the check was complete we would need to move cities at a few days' notice. In that short, too-lucid span of time, I had nothing to do. I hadn't yet found a new job. I'd finished a giant project for the synagogue, which had just moved into its first permanent home, the triumphant ending to an exhaustive and exhausting fourteen-year capital campaign. My days stretched out in front of me, empty, with every reasonable grown-up I knew heads-down in their offices.

And so I picked up the project of Warren again. Tentatively, by one corner. I didn't look any different, but constant exhaustion and nausea reminded me that I was making a new family, one that I hoped would be more stable than the original. With that shift in perspective, the project seemed more manageable. His absence no longer felt like a black hole, but like the shutter sealing off an old lead-paned window; something was on the other side, something was reachable. All it would take was muscling through.

I had no idea there was such a thing as a forensic genealogist. They contract out to probate firms, insurance companies, and military repatriation efforts, looking for missing debtors or missing heirs. I hired one I found on Yelp, a kindly woman named Leslie who searched through sheaves of official records I didn't even know existed.

She poked around on Ancestry.com and it was there that she came up with the grail: she found the profile of a woman named Lydia Grant who was connected to the Luther family. It had to be Warren's wife. Bingo. I thought back to the woman on the other end of the phone, who had denied knowing Warren, let alone being married to him; was this the same person?

If it was, she'd had a hell of a change of heart. Leslie reached out to her, saying only that she was doing research on behalf of "a family member" and verifying that she was in fact Warren's wife; Lydia replied, her tone measured and calm, saying she was happy to talk to Warren's relative. She was on Ancestry for the most prosaic of reasons, conducting her own search for her grandfather—a charming con man with, she suspected, a better story than her family would admit to. Would the relative like to reach out directly?

I reeled. Finally, a person who had not just known Warren, but presumably had loved him. Who had survived his suicide and rebuilt her life after him. Who knew more about him than a few months of sadness and *Sounds of Silence* on repeat, who might own more of him than a backgammon set of questionable provenance. Someone who would have memories of him, real ones, ones I could trust. Someone who had—as far as I was aware—no reason to lie to me. I put my head between my knees and breathed deep, trying to calm the hitch. Maybe it only works in movies. I felt like I was going to scream with joy, burst into hysterical weeping, or throw up. Or all three.

Before I could gather myself, another email appeared; the genealogist had forwarded it with the subject line "!!!"

"Hello, Liz," Lydia wrote.

Leslie Corn has told me that you are doing family research into the Crow family, including my father-in-law, Frank Luther (Crow) and would like to know something about his son, Warren Frank Luther. I am pleased to provide you with the information I have from my short connection with the Luther family.

Warren and I were married in New York City in October 1973. He was 25 then (born on August 11, 1948). I've attached a rather faded photo [Ed. note: A photo! A new photo!] of him taken in 1976—playing football in Central Park with a local team, a great joy of his. He was born at New York Hospital and lived his entire life in Manhattan. He went to the Collegiate School through high school and attended Syracuse University and Bard College, but didn't graduate from either. During our marriage, he worked as a loan counselor at a finance agency and also in the accounting department of the Saks Fifth Avenue department store. [So: Not AmEx. And nary a mention of a tour in Vietnam.]

He was highly intelligent, athletic, gregarious, attractive, and very, very sweet.

However, Warren was a very serious alcoholic—a problem that came to light after the first year of our marriage, when he could no longer hide it from me. As you may know, it is understood today that alcoholism is a disease, not a moral failing, and that it often runs in families. Warren told me (and his sister, Helen, confirmed) that his mother, Dorothy, was also an alcoholic, as were several members of her Canadian family. I don't believe that was true of the Crow family, although I only knew Frank Luther (Crow)— and he was not an alcoholic. He was seventy-four when I first met him. Warren told me his father had recently been diagnosed with "a cerebral atrophy." Based on my observations, I now believe that was a euphemism for dementia— possibly Alzheimer's disease. My father-in-law at that time was a totally delightful man whose memory was failing and who, several years after Warren and I were married, was moved to a nursing home, at least partly because of his tendency to "wander" late at night. (Warren's mother told us he had left their Manhattan apartment late one night in his underwear intending to "go to work.") Warren was devastated by his own inability to take care of his dad, whom he loved very much.

I paused and blinked tears furiously out of my eyes. After all these years, and after this terrible loss, Lydia was determined to convince a possibly unsympathetic stranger that Warren had been a good man in the grip of a hard life. How kind.

"When his mother learned of his death, she became despondent," she continued.

She called me numerous times to talk about him, but eventually was stopped from calling me by her daughter, who told me that her conversations with me were too depressing and that I was not to ever speak to her again. I didn't. I learned only years later that my mother-in-law died several months after Warren's death (in April 1978, I believe). I never learned how, but it would not surprise me if due to her overwhelming grief (and feelings of guilt that she expressed to me) she, too, took her own life. By that time, my father-in-law was in a nursing home. I don't know if they ever told him about these deaths. I later learned that he died in 1980.

I hope this information is useful to you. I would appreciate knowing how you are related to Warren and if you may have information about him or his immediate family that I don't have.

And there it was.

I closed the laptop and paced the room, my head blank and shrill. That relatively short email, which I'd speed-read in just a few minutes, contained at least ten times more information than I'd had in the thirty-seven years previous.

I sat down and read it again. And again.

A new line of communication had opened. I had to know more. The need was voracious; I felt like one of the zombies in *28 Days Later*, sprinting, teeth bared and slavering. My greatest fear was that not only would my existence come as a complete surprise to Lydia, but that my mother's would as well. What if the separation story had been a lie he had told her, or one my mother told me? Would I be giving her good news—that some part of Warren lived on? Or was I revealing his infidelity almost forty years later, when surely she had put her grief to rest?

And what if it wasn't real? What if she took a look at my picture and shook her head—no, you look nothing like him? What if she laughed and said, *Not after that vasectomy, you're not*? Now that I had my teeth in Warren's story, I wasn't sure I had it in me to start all over again with another father candidate.

I didn't want to deceive her. But I couldn't let her disappear, taking that first-last-and-only line of information with her. *Sound normal*, I instructed myself. *Don't scare her off*.

"Dear Lydia," I wrote, finally. "Thank you so much for all of the history you sent, and for your generosity in taking the time to write it all out for a perfect stranger. I have been trying unsuccessfully to find information on Warren's life for many years, and it feels like a miracle to have so much of it at once; I'm still processing it. You speak of him with such caring, even after what sound like some very tough years; I was so touched to read it, and I'm sorry to hear of the tragedies that followed so closely together.

"You asked how I am related to Warren. I'm struggling with how to word this, as I don't know if it will come as good news or bad, but I'm hoping it's good. In late 1977, Warren had a relationship with my mother, Judith Scheier. They didn't know each other long and she doesn't remember much (she also now has dementia), but she has told me that it was a relationship largely founded on mutual unhappiness—she was depressed, and I now understand from your email what a hard time he was going through. I was born in June 1978. I believe that Warren was my father."

I rubbed my burning eyes. *Stop looking for a good way to say this. There isn't one. You have to accept that you may be about to fuck up someone's memory of her dead husband. Don't sugarcoat it. Just convince her that at the very least, Warren's daughter isn't an asshole.*

"Lydia, I hope that this is good news and not upsetting news. Maybe it's not news at all. But in any case, I hope my contacting you has not reopened any old wounds, and I hope you know what a blessing it is for me to have some answers to questions that I thought would remain unanswered forever. If, after reading this, you would be willing to talk to me more about him—any stories that you have will be new to me—it would mean the world to me."

And I tapped out some closing pleasantries, and I hit send. And remembering the year and a half I spent haunting the mail for a picture, I settled down for a long wait.

She responded less than an hour later.

She was shocked, she said, but not upset. She knew about my mother. She and Warren had separated because of his drinking, and were both seeing other people, but always with an eye toward getting back together. He wanted to reconcile; she told him he could move back in, but that the first time he came home drunk, he would have to leave.

The night before he was to move back in permanently, he came home drunk. A test? An act of self-sabotage? Who knows?

She told him to leave. I don't know if there was an argument, or if he tried to convince her to let him in, or if he turned silently away. I don't know if she was surprised that he was drunk, or surprised that it took so long. But he left. He went upstairs to the roof of the building, and he clambered up over the railing, and he jumped.

They say that if you're looking for a surefire way to end

your own life, the most certain method is to jump off something high. You can stick the barrel of a gun in your mouth and pull the trigger, and end up with a shattered jaw. You can try to drown yourself and end up swimming back to shore, your body taking over where your mind shut down. Nooses snap, pills come back up as vomit, garages with running cars have unexpected drafts.

But jump off something high, and there's no net to catch you. No divine hand swoops out of the sky, palm upturned. It's just you and the air and the whistle and the smash.

His death certificate reads, under "Cause of Death": "Fractures of skull, ribs, pelvis, and extremities. Lacerations of internal organs. Fall from roof of residence, 520 E. 81st St." (I grew up at number 345 of the same street. Less than two blocks away.)

In layman's terms: everything broke.

He started with a young, strong, football player's body. He flung it off the roof of the building. Or maybe not flung: maybe dropped. Maybe he sat on the edge with his feet dangling, considering his options, and finally dug the heels of his hands against the concrete and pushed. Maybe he took it at a run, closing the distance between roof door and empty space in a few seconds.

The story did give me some information that came as a relief. I had always been afraid that it had been not a deliberate jump, but an accident. But no: he had left Lydia a note. At least he had not just leaned too far over the railing, watching the passersby below. At least he had gotten what he—at least at that moment—wanted.

They say that suicide is a permanent solution to a temporary problem. "Temporary" is doing a lot of work in that aphorism. Over the span of a (short) life, what's temporary? A week? A month? As many years as you can remember? When is enough too much?

Warren had been drinking his way out of his life since high school, Lydia told me, if not before. His mother drank herself unconscious through much of his childhood. Helen had told her how awful it had been to arrive home with a date, only to find her mother passed out on the floor. He and his classmates drank early and often. They had shitty home lives, and being drunk meant being somewhere else for a change. Why *not* forget? Why would you want to remember?

It's hard to blame him, and I don't—though that's easy for me to say. We don't ever have the full view of the desert of someone's despair.

I play the what-if game endlessly, futilely. What if he had lived? Would he and my mother have stayed together, their relationship suddenly and sharply given longevity via shared parenthood? Would he have reined my mother in, or served as a much-needed bridge to the outside world? Would she have curbed his drinking? Would he have taken the birth of his child as a catalyst to go to meetings, go inpatient, get help?

On the other end of the spectrum—the pessimist side that says this is all wish fulfillment—I started spinning out all the worst possible timelines. I imagined, with dread, a childhood filled not only with shrieking but with broken bottles, a father with alcoholism and a mother with borderline personality disorder playing off each other, her fear of abandonment fulfilled by his drunken absence. Or a suicide delayed instead of prevented, my mother left with a mourning child to top off her own grief.

Clearly I hadn't actually won the Shitty Family Olympics, just placed in the qualifiers. It could've been worse.

Lydia and I kept emailing, politely, and increasingly warmly. She'd had no one to talk to about him in years, and now here was a ravenous audience for every tiny detail she could dredge out of her memory. I wanted every fact, no matter how inconsequential. I was making up for lost time.

When I'd tried to imagine who my father might have been, I'd done some Universal Crappy Single-Parented Kid Math; I subtracted my mother from myself and conjured a person out of what was left. The math, I quickly saw, was wrong.

Warren Frank Luther was born Frank Daniel Luther. His mother, a consummate snob, thought better of the middle name they planned to use—"Every Irish bartender in New York is called Danny," she'd said (*And well she should know*, I thought unkindly)—and crossed out the original name on his birth certificate with a thick black line.

Like me, he grew up in Manhattan. But it was a different kind of childhood. His father, Frank Luther, was a well-known radio personality and children's entertainer. A close friend of Will Rogers and Gene Autry, he even has a star on the Hollywood Walk of Fame. He was a loving and cheerful man who spent most of his time out of the apartment and away from Dorothy, whose drinking was becoming more and more of a hazard.

She looked down on Warren's Catholic-raised wife too. "She's very sweet, dear, but she's not one of us," she told him after he'd brought Lydia home. Dorothy came to New York from Montreal to become an actress, and her wealthy father disowned her, bringing her back into the fold only when she quit acting to become a wife and mother. Drinking kept her from functioning as much of either, and she had the staff to step in—a nanny called "Doodles," a maid/cook, and a chauffeur.

(This last especially blows my mind—by the time I was growing up in New York, not one of my acquaintances knew how to drive or had a car to practice on. Driver's ed was a mysterious term I would have sworn was archaic, like home ec, and when I went to college I viewed my driving classmates with a mixture of wonder and distrust. I didn't learn to drive until my midtwenties, when all the drivers at my volunteering gig retired. Not only a car, but a *chauffeur*? What kind of family *was* this?)

Dorothy had a life-sized wooden giraffe sent from FAO Schwarz that had to be hoisted up the side of the building and in through a window, as it was too big to fit in the elevator. I thought of my own painfully awkward middle-school days haunting the aisles there. My mother had bought me dolls from the side register, where cut-price toys were available for sale to the nannies of wealthy families to give their charges as birthday gifts. Arie had been an extra in the movie *Big*, cast as an Orthodox yeshiva student on a field trip to the store with his class and rabbi, and was fitted with a tall hat and fake *payos*. The family eagerly awaited the release of the movie only to have the scene hit the cutting-room floor; someone luckily pointed out to the director, before the cut was finalized, that Orthodox Jews do not shop on Saturdays. So much for the Jewish-controlled media cabal, *nu*?

But Warren's family had shopped there. And they had paid *retail*. He might as well have dropped from Mars.

Lydia remembered him with an enormous amount of affection; an empathetic, outgoing young man with an over-supply of energy and love, burdened with an illness that was his undoing. Buried in that kind, accepting email is only one line that hints at the swerve she must have been feeling, the suddenly shifting sod under her feet. "I have always believed," she wrote, "(at least until I received your email) that if it were not for his alcoholism, we would be married today."

What did she mean by that quiet, sad parenthetical? Would she have found it too hard to take him back, knowing he had a child out there? Did she assume he would have left her for the mother of that child? Did the entrance of a whole other person into the mix just throw her memory into complete disarray, a variable that couldn't have been anticipated?

She sent pictures. In one he stands on a football field in Central Park, hands on hips, squinting into the sun. He wears a raglan-top shirt and has 70s shagged hair and sideburns. In another, he sits on a daybed piled with loud floral pillows under a batik wall hanging, a soft-stomached cat draped over his legs like a Dali clock. The photo is slightly out of focus, but he looks like the kind of man who would be fuzzy a foot in front of your eyes; his features are soft with youth, his expression untroubled. His soft blue eyes are blameless and wide set, lending the unnerving impression that you can't quite focus on both at once.

I'd had that same blunt nose and weak, soft chin, which sloped lumpily into my neck. A few hours in Dr. Magic Hands's office and a silicone implant remedied both. I'd assumed the nose was from somewhere back in the woodpile on my mother's side; who would have guessed that my prominent schnoz came from my goyische father?

A few days later, I got an email from the alumni rep from Warren's high school class in response to my query. Now that I had gotten a taste of Lydia's memories, the bit was between my teeth. If I could reconstruct some portion of his life from other people's narratives, I might be able to formulate something like a picture of him. Some understanding of who he had been.

I got on the phone with Robert in a not-yet-furnished office in our brand-new synagogue, sandwiched in between meetings. I sat cross-legged on the floor with my laptop balanced on my lap, plugged in my headset, breathed, dialed.

Robert's voice was warm, and he sounded genuinely thrilled to hear from me. No, he hadn't lived in New York in some time; he was now in California, working in film, where the sun shone all the time and he could spend time with his family. I tried to be as open-ended as I could: What had Warren been like?

"Warren was a great guy," he said immediately. "I came to Collegiate late; I was fifteen, and the rest of the class already knew each other. They assigned me to Warren as a 'shadow,' you know what I mean?" I did. "Someone to hang out with. I was really trepidatious about it—I was shy. But Warren was so full of life and personality, we just hit it off.

"We were in a band together. Warren played the drums, I played bass, two seniors played guitar. One guy named Gary, who lives in California now. And one guy named Kenneth—what? No, I have no idea how to get ahold of him. The band was called the Trees. He was a wonderful drummer. This would have been . . . what, 1964 or 1965. We played at schools, parties, charity events, we had fun, we got paid for it." He paused. "I'd already been drinking for a couple of years. Warren also liked to drink. But I guess you knew that."

"Yeah, I did. That's the reason he killed himself—he wanted to get sober and he couldn't."

"Oh. I see." I heard his palm move over his face. "I got sober in my thirties—I went to AA, it was much later, 1984. A lot of our friendship and bonding was over drinking together and smoking pot together." His voice was slightly bashful, in the way older people get when they talk to young people about boozing it up or getting high; I heard him remember that I was no spring chicken myself, and he went on with more confidence. "We'd go to a bar and have beers at lunchtime instead of eating lunch. He was a party. He was charming, full of life, everyone was drawn to him.

"And we played football together. He was a center, or a linebacker or something. He would puff himself up, pretend to be scary to intimidate the other team."

I laughed. "Was he a big guy?"

"Yeah, oh, yeah. All shoulders and back. Maybe five foot ten, dirty blond hair, pale complexion, teenage acne. Very strong. His father had an office on Fifty-Fifth between Park and Lex, around the corner from Central Synagogue—You know where that is? Good—we would hang out there and drink beer. We'd go to girls' apartments, you know, the old-money ones, and practice on the weekends. We played the Beatles and the Beach Boys. He had a real drummer personality—You know what I mean? No?—he was kind of a wild man, crazy, impulsive. We'd go to the Berlin Bar, drink sloe gin fizzes and Singapore slings."

I laughed. "Those sound to me like Hawaiian vacation drinks, not teenage boy drinks!"

"Yeah," he said thoughtfully. "We mostly just cared that they were strong."

When we got off the phone, he wrote to his class, asking them to send me memories. And did they ever. Their memories of that time in their lives were far clearer than any of my own. Many of them were wistful or outright melancholy. They had already lost a few of their number to either alcoholism or suicide or both. They were of an age when you don't yet consider yourself elderly, but neither does your obituary contain the word "tragic." The death of a classmate would have felt like someone walking over their grave.

"I have often thought of your dad over the years since high school," began one.

As twelve-year-olds after school, we would meet in an alley between two apartment buildings to smoke cigarettes and hang out. He smoked Winstons, which I moved up to after starting out on extremely mild Spring cigarettes and King Sano. That made us more equal and partners in hipness. Eventually we smoked Marlboros, making us Marlboro Men in our minds. We both came from difficult family situations, which neither of us discussed at the time but somehow sensed in one another and were therefore drawn to one another.

Your dad was also very intellectually curious and had a serious interest in history, especially World War II and the rise of Nazism. I remember him gaining the admiration of my father, who was an historian in his own right, when they chatted briefly about the war. I was again impressed because winning my father's admiration was never easy for me, especially in intellectual matters. [*Ugh*, I thought. *There's a story there.*]

Warren and I both played four years of varsity football. His locker room antics were hysterically funny. I remember him putting his football helmet on backward, resting atop his head, which gave the impression of his forehead rising upward like some Martian. He would howl out imitations of Soupy Sales and White Fang, an early 60s comedian and his dog. On the football field your dad was a ferocious player, frequently exhorting other players to push themselves harder to win. After one successful game, your father and I and two other players were MVPs and awarded tickets to a Jets game at Shea Stadium. At the game one of the other players brought a bottle of whiskey to warm us in the late fall weather. We passed the booze up and down the aisle to one another and had a good time. However, little did we realize that our coach and headmaster were sitting three rows behind us observing our every belt of liquor. We were all kicked off the team and the championship was lost.

In ninth grade or tenth, I believe, your dad became the drummer for the band the Trees, with Gary on lead guitar, Kenneth on rhythm guitar, and Robert on bass. Drums were the perfect instrument for Warren to pound out his pent-up feelings. At our frequent parties the booze and beer flowed freely and the music was loud and explosive. Your dad got to vigorously show off his skill with the drum solo in the song "Wipe Out." One time he got so carried away he fell over backward during the solo, right off his drumming stool. That was our nature in our adolescence—over the top.

Liquor was a big part of high school for many of us, not just with our peers but also in our families. For quite a few of us, drinking, in our families and in our own lives, was a source of our pain and a means of fleeing it. Because the drinking age was eighteen in New York at the time, we were able to hit the bars as early as the tenth grade. We had many a weekend of fun at the Gold Rail Tavern at 111th Street and Broadway, where we passed as Columbia University students and consumed pitchers of beer and glasses of Seagram's 7 and 7 Up. These were great times of friendly communion and a relief from the hard times some of us were experiencing in our homes. My father was a functioning and quite successful alcoholic, accomplished in his work, boundary crashing, sometimes hilariously so, abusive and sometimes violent in and out of the home. Your dad was experiencing something similar, I think, in his home.

One night your dad invited me and Paul over to his ground-floor apartment on East End Avenue to hang out. We were visiting in his bedroom with the door closed when suddenly we heard his mother, your grandmother, shriek in an alcohol-infused rage from the living room, "Waaaaaarren! Get those fucking kikes out of my house!" She screamed that repeatedly and the three of us boys climbed out the bedroom window into the grassy courtyard behind the apartment. As we escaped and headed up East End toward my house, your dad, who was walking between me and Paul, hung his head into the palms of his hands in shame and embarrassment and sobbed. Such pain was familiar to all of us and we passed no judgment on your dad.

Many of us in our class had tough family situations, but we rarely talked about it or had the skills to do so. In some ways we were trapped in a school situation which demanded rigorous academic achievement while ignoring the deeper issues we were facing. Some of us found relief with girlfriends in our first loves. Others relied on drink or pot to help us through. Though no idiot, I managed to graduate at the very bottom of my class, but because of Collegiate School's reputation, I was able to get into the University of Wisconsin on a phone call. Your dad to his great credit was a much better student and was admitted to Syracuse University, no small feat.

We lost touch after high school, but were he alive today, I would so love to reconnect with your father. He was a bright, talented, funny, passionate, and compassionate human being, a truly special person. I have thought of and missed him many times over the years and can only imagine your sorrow in not having had him in your life. He would be so grateful and proud of you for seeking out who he truly was.

I read the story and laughed uneasily, fingering the Star of David I wore around my neck. Well. That's one relationship I didn't need to miss, then. The ultimate revenge against the rampant anti-Semite: the Jewish mistress, the observant daughter. Mom and I looked like WASPs, but we were two generations off the boat and one step ahead of the camps. Dorothy would have hated us. I gave my long-dead grandmother a mental middle finger.

The thought of Warren being proud of me was a bit of an electric shock. As a kid I had indulged in plenty of fantasies of him sweeping me away, adoring of his child; it had never occurred to me to consider our relationship as adults. Of course, by the time Tom's email arrived, I was a decade older than Warren ever got. I didn't like to think that I was getting a leg up on a parent in terms of maturity.

So: What did I learn?

My erstwhile father was, of all things, a football player. A drummer. A teenage bon vivant, a college dropout, a charmer, an entertainer, an alcoholic.

The high school friends remembered him as the biggest guy in the room, the guy with the loudest laugh, slamming the biggest beer. I kept coming back to the story of his floppy-haired self slapsticking backward right off his drum stool. I mean. You've got to love a guy like that.

They sent me scans of the yearbook. His photos show a young man with hair so neat you can see the comb marks, the familiar cowlick twisting up the side. He is blowing smoke rings at the camera. He crouches with a football helmet on his knee, squinting into the camera. He poses in a stunt picture over a pile of bricks from the school's ongoing construction project, wagging a piece of pipe at another student. Knowing what I know now, it's clear from his expression that he—like many of the students in the photo, taken at midday with the sun glaring overhead—is drunk.

Most of the stories the Collegiate class had to tell me took place in the bars. He'd played pool at a Seventy-Ninth Street pool hall—the one where I sank halfhearted eight balls in high school? Who knew? Music, always music, and the gleeful knowledge that they were not fighting in the Vietnam War. Years later, he told my mother that he had served. Or she made it up. Or she forgot that it wasn't true. Or she convinced herself that it was.

Lydia had never remarried. I didn't ask why. I struggled hard with the knowledge that she didn't know me at all and owed me nothing, and that, at the same time, she was the only living person in the world who could tell me who he had really been as an adult. The only way I had to eke out this long-awaited information—the only way to assuage my own sadness—was to surface a painful past for someone else.

I never did figure out the right balance. Lydia and I discovered a mutual love for theater and traded recommendations; when I moved to DC, we met for an eerily blind date–esque lunch, and talked about travel, our families, her search for her grandfather. We didn't mention Warren at all. We kept up an occasional email correspondence, a few times a year, movies and books and general chat. When my second child was born, middle-named Warren as per Jewish tradition for the dead, she wrote back with great grace: "Congratulations on your beautiful baby boy. (His name touches me deeply.) All the best to your beautiful family."

I wondered if she thought of me as the ghost ship that hadn't carried her, the daughter she might, under less tragic circumstances, have had. If my children were the grandchildren she didn't get to spoil. I kept our conversation focused on the positives and the joys. I was too shy to ask her many more questions about Warren. I didn't want my fireball of all-consuming need to scare or spook her. She had been through enough.

Before Arie and I left New York, I crossed the road behind the Met and sat on a step overlooking Turtle Pond under Belvedere Castle, where I now knew Lydia had spread Warren's ashes. The pond and the whole area had been revitalized years before, not long after the premiere of *Pocahontas* on the Great Lawn—rumor had it Disney had ponied up for the revitalization in exchange for the opportunity to screen the movie there—and I knew that there was no more trace of him in that water or in that earth. But I sat anyway, and I talked to him. I told him about the overlaid maps of our lives, all taking place in the same few square miles of the city. I told him about tracking down his ashes, and about the unnerving meeting at Frank E. Campbell, and about Lydia's scrawled signature on the crematorium's form. I told him what his high school classmates remembered about him. I told him I wished he'd stuck around, but that I understood why he hadn't. I told him I was sorry that I was leaving. I told him Lydia missed him. I told him I did too.

And I stood up, and I brushed off my butt, and I bought an overpriced ice cream sandwich and ate it in three bites on the way out of the park. It took almost forty years, but I had finally visited my father's grave. Turtles and all.

CHAPTER 10

Hitched

The younger dimwit cat, afraid of everything bigger than a dust mote and sometimes those, too, refused to eat the tranquilizer treat before getting in the car. The genteel old-lady cat obliged, and while Pisa scratched and panted in a carrier at my feet, Elvis sat contentedly in my diminishing lap as we drove away from Brooklyn, paws on the window frame, watching the highway spool by. They both looked calmer than I felt. Except for college, I had never lived outside New York, and leaving it felt unreal. John Updike was right when he said, "The true New Yorker secretly believes that people living anywhere else have to be, in some sense, kidding."

With every mile that passed, I breathed a little easier. Mom had responded to the news of the move with characteristic panic and anger, and the growing distance between the car and her apartment felt as figurative as it did literal. I had stopped sending her money when I lost my job, and she seemed to be managing just fine. I took a deep breath and rolled my skull back and forth against the headrest, relieved.

I was three months pregnant, engaged to a man, and about to move to a city with hundreds of politicians and zero publishing industry. One of my favorite mental games is to go back in time and tell my mopey twenty-year-old self where I am now, gleefully watching her surprise; I updated her silently and watched her spontaneously combust.

We settled into a small, nondescript apartment in DC and I promptly got a job at a nonprofit, where I wore loose-fitting pants to hide my stomach. After a lifetime in New York, DC felt like a city designed by Disney. It's small—even the most generous definition of the metro area doesn't bring it to the million-occupant mark—and transient, as people move in for administrations and then back out when a new one comes in. In fairness, we were at a sedate stage of life. We were approaching middle age and I was pregnant. If there were orgies happening in our building, no one was inviting us anyway.

We went home to New York to get married. There's something to be said for being five months pregnant at your own wedding. Quite a bit, actually. Wedding planning takes a backseat to doctor's appointments, dress options are narrowed down considerably, and you can eat a diner platter of chocolate chip pancakes the size of a hubcap for pre-wedding brunch without worrying about bloating. Claire and I sat in a Sixth Avenue diner, chatting and kicking our feet against the high-set booth. I tried to get her to try my egg cream. It took all of her Midwestern politeness to say no nicely.

The photographer trailed around after us as I got my face made up and airbrushed (yes, this is a thing) and my hair done up and as Claire zipped me into the practical empire-waist white J. Crew dress I'd gotten on eBay. It turns out if you throw a wedding at a hotel, they give you a deal on a suite where you can host friends for pizza the day before, a set of Broadway-themed rooms with signed playbills on the walls ("*It's Patti fucking LuPone!*" I gasped, and the young photographer nodded politely, no idea at all who I was so excited about) and leopard-spotted throw rugs tossed jauntily over tufted velvet couches. ("You look like you're wearing a Muppet," scolded a friend when I tossed one faux-elegantly around myself.) I took a bath, I admired my pedicured toes, I winked at myself in the round mirror positioned coyly over the bed. A pregnant wedding is a sober wedding, and I was alert for every moment of it.

When it was time, Claire and I crossed Thirtieth Street in a haze of August heat, my dress hiked around my knees to keep it from dragging in the street. Passersby yelled jovial congratulations. We sneaked upstairs to the hallway outside the synagogue balcony; Arie was holding his *tisch* downstairs. Our friends and family surrounded him, eating dry kosher cookies and mainlining seltzer and roasting him roundly. The photographer caught some fantastic moments—old friends greeting each other enthusiastically; his parents laughing, heads together; our old friend Yumi hamming it up, arm sweeping exaggeratedly overhead to demonstrate the "world's longest movie-theater yawn" move as twenty-five years of friendship turned to love.

One photo in particular has stuck with me. In the foreground a clutch of our friends are catching up, hands on each other's arms and shoulders. In the far corner my mother sits alone. She is slumped slightly in her chair, sacklike dress pooling at her midsection. I recognize her expression—head tilted, eyes focused in the middle distance, like someone put her in power-save mode. She's lonely, and she feels abandoned. Which she had been, kind of. Tor and his wife had volunteered to get her dressed and out of her apartment to the synagogue, but they couldn't be expected to take the sharp side of her tongue every moment. Looking at the picture, I still hear my lizard brain snap at me, *Go*—go talk to her, entertain her, fix it. The Mother of the Bride needs company and you are *delinquent.*

These are the moments I found hardest during that eventful year. No amount of effortful pragmatism could keep me from wanting the Movie Moments. I know that not everyone gets the sweet mother-daughter bonding moments over the wedding stuff and the pregnancy stuff, but I felt their absence keenly. She should have clipped me into sample dresses, shedding happy tears into her complimentary champagne when we found The One. She should have sat up with me the night before, giving me marriage advice, either wise or hilarious—"leave the gun, take the cannoli," Caitlin's mother had told her sagely, tapping the side of her nose. I should have called her for a calm-down when vendors flaked out or things went wrong. I should have run the ketubah language by her. I should have sent her every ultrasound photo, even the twenty-week monstrosity we called "Skeletor," where Rachel bared tiny half-formed jaws in the direction of my heart.

I didn't do any of that. I couldn't. Having a mentally ill parent meant simultaneously wrestling with a hard relationship while mourning the absence of the one you actually wanted. I wanted *a* mother to clip me into those dresses, but not *my* mother. Someone who would tell me I looked beautiful without staring at me hungrily, as if she wanted to subsume me. Someone who could keep her fury in check, who wouldn't smash her champagne glass on the floor if the attendant said something she didn't like. Aren't there companies in Japan that will rent you a stand-in boyfriend for a wedding? Where's the rental stand-in for mother of the bride? Couldn't capitalism throw me a bone here?

When Caitlin arrived she snuck upstairs and found me in the hallway, where I was nervously pacing, my heels piled in a corner. The last time we'd seen each other was almost exactly a year before, when I'd wept on her porch trying to figure out why Laura was leaving. She grabbed me in a giant hug and lifted me, pregnant belly and all. "*Well*, Scheier," she said. "This year has *rather* turned around."

Someone cleared his throat, and we turned around. Torsten, who'd been chaperoning my mother, was standing there looking slightly sick.

"So don't shoot the messenger," he said.

"Jesus." I put my hand on my hips, bent forward, breathed deeply. "What?"

"Your mother says she's walking you down the aisle."

I straightened up and shook my head, uncomprehending. "No, I told her we're each walking alone. Does she not remember that we talked about this?"

He shifted, clearly wanting to be anywhere but here. "She remembers, but she doesn't care. She says she's walking you down the aisle or she'll stand in the middle of it and block your way."

So.

I should have known. I should have *fucking* known that there was no moment too personal to ruin, nothing she considered outside of her purview. Somewhere in the white tulle–wrapped depths of my soul, I heard one of the last fibers of the rope binding me to her snap.

"Listen. I'm sorry you got stuck in the middle of this. But please go down and tell her no one's walking either of us down the aisle. We're walking by ourselves. OK?"

He nodded and fled. It was four o'clock; time for the ceremony to start. Claire held my hand, rubbed my sequined back. "Only your mother," she said glumly.

"I'm almost forty years old, I'm not having my damn mother walk me down the aisle!" I fumed. The rabbi appeared.

"So, we seem to be having some trouble with your mom." I dropped my head and groaned. "She wants to come upstairs and see you, and says that she will disrupt the whole ceremony if you say no. I want you to know that I will support *whatever you want to do*. If you want to allow her to do this, we can bring her up. If you want her in the wedding, we can rearrange the procession, no problem. If you say no and she causes a scene, security can escort her out of the building and keep her there. *Whatever you want.* OK?"

Downstairs, my mother started screaming.

A part of me—a very large part—wanted to tell the rabbi to have my mother frog-marched out by security. I was so furiously tired of her weaponized anger, of the tantrums that got her whatever she wanted because I feared the scenes she could create. I didn't want to reward my mother's shitty behavior. But the downstairs was filled with our whole community, including Arie's whole extended family, who barely knew me and knew nothing of her history.

She had me backed into a corner, and she knew it. If I held

firm, the story of my marriage would start with That Time Liz Got Her Mother Arrested. The only way out was to give her what she wanted.

"OK," I said. "She can come up." The rabbi peered into my eyes, hugged me fiercely, and went down the stairs, my friends on her heels.

I stood alone, shoulders slumped. I hadn't imagined a zen-like, meditative state in these last moments before I got married. I'd imagined something more relaxed, more silly than holy. We'd forgone a wedding party, feeling too old to need a procession of people waiting for us at the bimah. Our parents were—were *supposed* to be—seated in the front row, craning their necks to see their children coming down the aisle. Our dearest friends were waiting outside the sanctuary holding the folded chuppah, surreptitiously checking their watches. And I was upstairs alone, trying to keep the world from finding out how fucked up my family was, and how huge my anger was. She also wanted that Hallmark Channel mother-daughter relationship. She also had ideas about how things were supposed to be, and about what a normal wedding send-off would be. She wanted to zip me into my dress and push bobby pins into my hair and clasp a something-new around my wrist. But failing all that she would settle for being the last person to see me before the wedding, and if that meant shouting down the house, she'd do it.

The screaming cut off. There was a brief, blessed silence. The tiny elevator dinged softly and my mother stepped out on Torsten's arm. Her hair was flattened back and her mascara-smeared eyes were huge, and I thought of a meerkat standing high, trembling, surveying the prairie. She came toward me, hands outstretched. "*Eliiiiiiizabeth*. You look so beautiful! I knew you would. I just wanted to see you."

I let her hug me, my arms stiffly at my sides, although her familiar perfume nauseated me and all I wanted to do was shove her away. "Thank you," I said through gritted teeth. "But you are disrupting the wedding ceremony. You are holding everyone up. Can you please go downstairs and sit down?"

"Yes, yes, of course!" she said jovially, as if I'd asked her to scoot down a seat to make room for a late arrival. She patted my hand. "Such a beautiful bride." Tor smiled at me, resigned, and I smiled back. He got her back on the elevator. I turned to find the wedding coordinator waiting at my elbow. "Do you need a minute?" she asked gently.

"No," I said. "Let's not waste any more time." I shook my head like a wet terrier, forcing her out of my mind. The wedding coordinator smoothed my hair back down, gently. And I went downstairs to get married.

Years later I watched our wedding video and kept it playing past the recession. Arie and I were downstairs in *yichud*, the tradition-mandated seclusion following the ceremony, where the married couple face each other alone for the first time. (Some people have sex. We chugged water and wolfed down cookies and laughed in hysterical, frenzied relief as Kat, our *yichud* guard, stood ramrod straight outside the door.) The string quartet is playing a bright major-key movement, and you can't hear anyone's individual voice over the music and the explosion of chatter, relieving the solemnity of the ceremony. Our friends collapse the chuppah, hug their spouses, greet late arrivals. And from the far right corner of the screen comes my mother, making a beeline for the rabbi. The rabbi puts a consoling hand on her arm; she swats it off. The Bodyguard

Friends approach, hover anxiously. She has on her Elderly Jewish Curmudgeon Persona face, brow furrowed and lips tight, and she gestures accusingly between herself and the rabbi. The rabbi's rainbow-kippahed head nods sympathetically, constantly, rabbinical bobblehead. The video fades out, and my sympathy with it.

CHAPTER 11

That's Why They Call It Labor

I went into labor at my desk.

I was working through lunch, and my distended, alien-queen stomach spasmed. I looked distrustfully down. The baby had already been gleefully kicking the strained muscles under my rib cage, and my whole midsection ached 24/7. It was hard to tell if this was something different.

I paced the apartment restlessly all night, my body spasming at random. By early the next morning we were sure it was go time. We spent the next hours watching TV and endlessly debating when to call the doula, who was going to drive us to the hospital. I'd been leery of hiring a doula—the whole setup reeked of patchouli and performative unmedicated labor—but my one-kidneyed self was high risk, and if I had to go in for emergency surgery, we wanted someone there to stay with the baby while Arie came with me. We didn't yet know anyone in

Washington well enough to invite them over to brunch, let alone our daughter's birth.

There was a snowstorm coming, and we decided to err on the side of caution. The doula arrived in a minivan with a dream catcher breezing from the rearview mirror, and I rolled my eyes through the pain. I hoisted myself into the passenger's seat. We chatted awkwardly, and every time a new contraction came, I grabbed the seat and yelled.

She stopped the car at a stop sign and looked for crossing traffic. And looked. And looked. And then stared straight ahead.

Long seconds passed, and I *awoogah*-ed through another contraction. No response.

Arie leaned forward. "Amanda?"

No response. She stared into the windshield, eyes glassy.

I looked at her, wild-eyed, and poked her in the leg. "*Amanda.*"

She came back to life, shuddered, and pulled into the intersection as if nothing had happened. I met Arie's eyes in the rearview mirror. He shook his head slightly.

When we arrived at the hospital, I slid out of the front seat with so much haste I almost went down in the slick of snow that had already started to fall. Pregnant women were lined up on a bench right inside the hospital entrance—clearly not dilated enough to be admitted, but as anxious about the snow as we were—and men paced in front of them, yelling into cell phones. Arie took my arm.

"What the *fuck*," I hissed.

"I think she had a petit mal seizure," he said grimly. "Just go. Worry about her later." She had pulled away to park, humming cheerfully.

She had a few more over the course of that long labor, the nurses navigating delicately around her as she stood stock-still with her palms facing stiffly forward, staring into space, and on one memorable occasion, she farted loud and long. We needed something to laugh about. Even with the blessed, blessed epidural it was many more hours of exhausting, red-faced work before Rachel slid into Arie's and the doctor's waiting hands. I was wearing the Labor Tiara that Arie had bought for me, mostly-not-really as a joke. I was tired and scared and—after reluctantly agreeing to let them bring a mirror so I could watch the progress—horrified by the sight of my body splitting open. But there she was, tiny and sweet and warm. "OH MY GOD," I said loudly, and then "Hi, sweetheart," and then, fervently, "Oh thank GOD I'm not pregnant anymore."

I didn't bond with her immediately. I felt like I'd been hit by the proverbial bus. I'd hated every moment of being pregnant. More than hated—resented. I was consumed with the feeling that this was the world's worst workflow; how on earth, in 2017, was the best way we had of making more people to *grow them inside existing people*? It boggled the mind. What about eggs and nests? What about incubators? How on earth have we not yet come up with a better way of doing this? Why women? Why *me*?

Those first few weeks passed in a fog. She slept—no, haha, obviously not slept, *spent her nights*—in a co-sleeper, a miniature crib pulled up next to my side of the bed, and every ninety minutes she woke up and wailed to be fed. I brought her into the living room, snapped the breastfeeding pillow around my waist, and latched the little piranha on. The whole production lasted a good forty-five minutes, and by the time I got her back to sleep, we had maybe half an hour before she woke up again. I don't think I went into REM sleep once in that first month.

There's a reason sleep deprivation is used as an interrogation tactic. I started having panic attacks where I swam up from blank, oven-hot sleep, certain that I was suffocating. Even once technically awake, I gulped for air and fumbled frantically at my throat. I bumped into furniture and apologized to doorways. Showering before noon was a rare victory, and when I did, I laid Rachel down on a towel on the bathmat, where she shrieked at me for the three miserable minutes it took to wash myself.

The whole world took on a surreal quality. I wasn't sure what was going on around me. But I knew I didn't like it. I tended to the baby every moment, but I felt no connection to her, nor to anything else.

Until. When Rachel was a few weeks old, she broke out in baby acne that covered her poor tiny face like smallpox. Cradling her in my lap, I thought about the horrors of middle school, of how other kids might tease her if she got zits, or was overweight, or whatever other minor infraction might bring down the Wrath of the Pubescent. And I was filled with a homicidal rage at this hypothetical band of brats that consumed me and filled me with incandescent anger. Anyone who was mean to her, I would kill. Slowly. And painfully.

And with that surge of righteous maternal fury, she was mine.

My mother wrote me a letter on my first birthday. "Incredible Child," she begins, and goes on to tell the story of my first year.

This time last year you were—well, honestly, a pretty dreadful ache inside me, struggling to be free. My reading and child-birth classes were for naught; tho' you chose to come early into the world—not expected till the 19th—perhaps you thought better of it, and slowed your progress to reconsider your haste out of the womb, for I did labor for 20 hours to bring you forth; having been told you'd be a "breakfast baby" at midnight, I hoped to hold you in my arms by 8 a.m., but you were then still high under my ribs, as if seeking shelter there, and, having pushed for over 7 hours, 3 of them with you crowning, it was with amazement and surprise that I beheld you, at 3:15 in the afternoon in a stream of sunlight, rosy red with bright blue hands and feet. How funny you looked! And I waited fully half an hour before allowing the cord to be cut; you nursed during that time, and so the circle was complete, you suckling at my breast, the cord stretching, now thin at having lost its function, between your body and mine. I felt so strongly that we should spend the rest of our lives, you and I, reaching for your independence, moving apart as it were, and so I begged for but a little more time for us to be one.

I could not then know that first we would spend much time growing together, reaching for each other in ways great and small, that each move you made toward being your own person, a being apart, would entwine our lives together in ways infinitely more binding than the cord which then seemed so fragile and useless a link. That you would possess me of such gladness and intimacy of spirit as I have never before known.

. . . Right, so. *Just* in case there was any confusion, my mother was not a Victorian maiden waxing rhapsodic to a schoolgirl correspondent, but a thirty-nine-year-old acerbic

Jew from Queens. Where this language came from—the laboring to bring me forth bit, et cetera—I couldn't begin to tell you.

And that is . . . *quite* a birth story, isn't it? Pushed for seven hours! I was approaching four hours when the team started prepping me for a C-section, concerned about Rachel's oxygen levels. Either she wiggled the right way or I heaved harder, because at the 3:57 mark she slid out into Arie's shaking hands. Talk about last minute; this is a kid who's always going to be doing her homework on the bus. Seven hours? I mean, not to call a new mother a liar. But.

I love that my mother begins with talking about that particularly intimate moment—when newborns cling to their mothers' skin, pissed about the light and the sound and trying to pick up something familiar—to start talking about our separating, something she never actually managed in real life. Truly, the lady is protesting too much, eh? But it's a good thought. She knows she's supposed to be helping me grow up and out. She's trying.

Motherhood puts you in the public eye in a way I found initially funny, then infuriating, then both funny and infuriating. When out for a walk with a hoodied newborn Rachel wrapped up under my winter coat, a man bellowed, "Lady! Put a fucking hat on that fucking baby!" (To my credit, I did *not* yell back, "Take some fucking anger management courses!") Women on the Metro advised me regarding my taste in onesies (anything hand-me-down), my phone (in existence and too close to the baby), and my shoes (high heels not being, in their view, appropriate for stroller-pushing). Every single day that I pushed my empty stroller the one block between the office and daycare for pickup, some wag—usually a man—

stopped me on the street and yelled some cheerful version of "Oh no! You forgot the baby!" I smiled stiffly, and deep down in my heart I sharpened my knives.

My husband, on the other hand, was treated like a cross between the most brilliant, self-sacrificing man on earth, and a performing monkey. When he walked into a Metro car wearing Rachel in a carrier, six people would leap up to offer their seats. Older women adjusted Rachel's hat, or held their hands surreptitiously up under her butt in case he dropped her. "Excuse me, sir," fluttered a woman in line at the grocery store, after we'd had our son. "I just wanted you to know that this is the best parenting I've ever seen. And I'm a pediatrician. I see a lot!" To earn this accolade (with which I don't disagree he deserves, but *come on*) he had kissed Rachel on the top of her head while singing to David his signature ballad, "David Is the Mayor of Babytown," a fairy-tale town in which houses go uncleaned, fires unfought, and garbage uncollected, because "babies just play all day"; you can sing endless stanzas to this song, describing a town riven with filth, burning to the ground, populated by feckless, cheery infants doing fuck-all with their days.

It's a low bar, is what I'm saying.

And all of this was nothing compared to pregnancy, of course. I worked in an office of a hundred or so people, and during each of my two pregnancies at least ten of them commented on my body every single day; near the end, it was always some variation of "Are you sure it's not twins ahahaha," and any time right before or after I delivered, it was "You don't even look like you're pregnant!" "You look so uncomfortable!" "You don't even look like you had a baby!" "You're so big!" "You're so small!" and my favorite, from a slight, well-intentioned gay man who grasped my elbows earnestly upon my return from having David: "This is just like last time! You look like it never even happened! Liz: *you did it!*" with the starry-eyed hero worship of a day hiker meeting Sir Edmund Hillary. I wasn't aware that there had been an *it* for me to *do*; I was just trying to cram in enough calories to keep my hands from shaking, as everything I ate seemed to be turning into buttercream for my Hulk of a baby.

I know they meant it kindly. I'm an American woman in the twenty-first century. It's my job to be thin, and if I've done it, especially in the aftermath of a body-wrenching, infrastructure-rearranging gig like pregnancy, the approval of my peers is my reward. But I just wanted to carry around an electric fly swatter and take a swing at anyone who spoke to me about how big or small I was, or how much I was or wasn't like I was before. I couldn't figure that out myself.

The loudest voices those years were pushing the idea of a "natural" childbirth, as if the other option was to produce a baby constructed of aspartame and Red #4. The vague, unspecified "natural" could mean anything at all: vaginal birth vs. C-section, unmedicated vs. epidural, spontaneous labor vs. induced. For women of a certain socioeconomic class and who feel generalized guilt about everything they do or fail to do, doing everything "naturally" became a competition and an exercise in self-abnegation, even if there was nothing at all natural about it. One woman I know had a "lotus birth," where instead of cutting her child's deflated umbilical cord, she allowed it to disintegrate off the child's body by itself, still attached to the rotting placenta, over the course of the first few days of the baby's life. "White nonsense," sneered an Indian friend, unimpressed by the "lotus" business.

I found myself drifting the other way, and fast. I mean, I

was careful. The only alcohol I drank during both pregnancies combined was a sip each of my friend's flight of three beers at my sober-for-me bachelorette party, and a half-glass of champagne to toast the speakers at my wedding. I kept the caffeine to a minimum, eschewed lunch meat and sushi, and, after a sample of soft cheese was literally slapped out of my hand by an overeager supermarket employee, gave up cheese. Without beer or coffee, I thought, I had no natively installed personality at all; the whole was constructed out of alcohol and caffeine. I curtailed my eating and drinking habits, refused cold medication, and snorked my way through a winter's worth of untreated workplace gunk.

But I *bitched*. Oh man, did I bitch. Soft-focus maternity shoot with our hands clasped lovingly over my bulging stomach? *Nope*. I rotated through a handful of funereally dark maternity dresses and increasingly insufficiently high-waisted maternity pants, and showed the pain I felt every time I stood up or sat down. Cheery attitude? *Absolutely not*. I answered all kindly queries with a bright "Just terrible, thanks! Pregnancy is the worst!" Pinterest-worthy nesting? *Ha. Ha. Hahahahahaha*. I was lucky enough to have a critical mass of friends who were finishing up their kid-having at just the right time, so I gratefully accepted enough hand-me-downs to get me almost to kindergarten ("Ask your mommy why she dresses you like a boy!" a daycare teacher prompted a bemused ten-month-old Rachel, who grabbed for her scarf and hooted) and belatedly hung some vaguely child-appropriate prints in the nursery.

Levelheaded Arie—unconcerned with public opinion—was an excellent foil for all of this. When for the hundredth day in a row I wept into Rachel's tiny head as she savaged my nipple trying to get out some of my woefully inadequate supply of milk, he put his arm around me. "I know you've been trying so hard to make this work," he said kindly. "But you do so many more important things for this baby every day than milk."

I didn't *Office Space* my breast pump into a field after that, but I did give up breastfeeding immediately, to all of our relief.

I needed that perspective. It helped that he was calm and careful about decision-making, but it mostly just helped to have another, different person opining on what the fuck we should be doing with this alien little person. I was totally out of my depth. I wondered how anyone could entrust me with a cactus, let alone an infant. I needed someone to bounce ideas off, and to tell me that I was doing fine.

My heart ached, unexpectedly, for my mother. In this same situation, she had been alone. Not just alone as in single, or alone as in without family, but alone in a world that moved differently than she did. She had been fearful and fierce, adoring and protective. She was obsessed rather than besotted. Her love sat squarely on my chest, obstructing my breathing.

This was my greatest fear: that I would be a mother like she was.

This is now my greatest fear: That by rearing back from that possibility, I'll go too far in the other direction. That I won't know the difference between saving my children from poisonous, overweening love, and keeping my feelings for them so tempered that they don't see them at all. That I'll overcompensate so much that they feel abandoned. I don't trust myself to love them the right amount.

Don't we all fear becoming our parents? They're embedded in us, enraged as it may make us. Impossible to purge the turns of phrase. Impossible to shed the muscle memory of gesture. This stuff sticks and sticks tight.

I wasn't frightened for my kids' safety the way so many of my friends were. I wasn't scared that I'd eaten too many nitrates, or of traces of caffeine hiding in an iced tea, or of fumes or parabens or toxins. I don't fear kidnappers, and I've never even glanced at the National Sex Offender Registry. While Arie would pace the floor with a feverish baby, waiting anxiously for the on-call doctor to phone, I'd get the cold washcloth, but I wouldn't worry. "She's fine," I'd say impatiently, and not a little smugly. "Babies get fevers. What's the worst that could happen?"

The worst has already failed to happen. I have not turned into my mother. Yet. Maybe ever.

But still, for every day I spend with them, the hamsters on the wheel in my head race without stopping. I test my every motion and comment and expression for sanity. Is this what a normal mother says or does? How about *this*? I do a complicated calculus of how close to hold them and how often to say "I love you." I try to strike the right balance between making sure they know they are perfectly, eternally loved, and giving them some damn space. I realize this is not rational. I do it anyway.

This still isn't instinctive for me. I don't know how to be a mother without being a net. Not the kind stretched taut to catch you if you fall, but the kind that drops on you, corners weighted, from the trees.

I rarely thought about the children who were born from my donated eggs until I had my own. Or, more accurately, until I had my second. My daughter favors me, blond and yellow skinned, and my son looks just like his father, his uncle, and his grandfather: olive skin, gentle, close-set eyes, a giant smile. But mostly they look like each other. They fight plenty, generally when we've made the rookie mistake of only having one of a toy. (One day I came home to find them happily tossing potatoes into the air; "Listen," Arie said wearily, "I needed something we had an even number of.") But they adore each other, and when they tumble across the floor together like baby weasels, shrieking and giggling, the ever-present knot in my heart loosens and I start to think: Maybe this will be OK. Even if I turn out to be like my mother, they will have each other. They will be safe.

And when I see them running around like tiny perpetual-motion machines, shrieking with happiness, I think: there are more of you.

I don't feel strongly connected to those mystery children. I certainly don't feel, as some traumatized donors do, that I have given my children to another woman to raise. I am not their mother in any sense but the genetic. They have a mother, or mothers, or fathers.

But they *are* my children's half-siblings.

So. What do you do?

After a lot of deliberation, I joined the Donor Sibling Registry. The registry looks to connect siblings born of a mutual sperm or egg donor, or genetic parents and children. I have very little information about my donations; just dates of retrieval (only because of the dated checks) and the name of the clinic. I called the clinic and got my donor number, which may or may not have ever made it to the intended parents. I also asked for my records, which arrived with some significant redactions; there are records of the follicles spotted by ultrasounds, and of my hormone levels at various points throughout the cycle, but there are no records of my dosages, and no records of the number of eggs retrieved. Gamete donors are specifically carved out from HIPAA protections, and I have no legal rights to my records. Technically, I'm lucky they gave me anything at all.

I haven't done DNA testing. I'm fearful of what I'd find if I dug too deep, to uncover yet another trail of lies. On my mother's scale of lying, anything is possible. I might find out that Warren had a passel of other children, or that my mother did not, in fact, have any.

There is apparently a line up to which I desperately want the truth and have difficulty tamping down my rage at not getting it, or at being deliberately deceived. But past that line—I can't take anymore. Past that line, I can't do another upheaval. I am willing to find out that Warren had a liking for coke, that my mother launched an ill-fated boutique law firm, that she *schtupped* every man in sight. All fine. But I don't know that I can take news of more siblings, or of a second missing genetic parent. There is only so much shock I can process, and I am drained.

When David was still an infant, I wrote to an editor who I knew from my publishing days to congratulate her on the publication of a new book on motherhood, a book that spoke with blistering honesty about how new mothers disappear from public lives and too often from their own. How our exhaustion and our hormones and our newly disordered lives keep us quiet, keep us distracted, keep us headed home early. She had recently adopted a toddler, and I had two; we were both in the weeds. I thanked her for shepherding into the world a book that I so badly needed. It was a relief to see my own thoughts reflected, not the blissed-out, loving haze of early parenthood, but the grief at the narrowing of my life that was the inevitable effect of its deepening, my blind anger at the systems, biological and societal, rigged so badly against women. "YES," she wrote back.

"I felt betrayed the whole first year. You are a different person but everyone expects you to be the person you were."

This wasn't what I felt. I *was* the same person—more tired, more easily frustrated, and tied to a newly restricted schedule, but still yearning for the social connection and mental stimulus I could no longer have. I still loved travel, but knew this was years away in our future; I still lived for books, but could find only a few minutes at a time to read them. I was not a different person. I was the same person, with two new loves, and no time or headspace to pursue the old ones.

There's a wonderful scene in the last season of *Orange Is the New Black*. Our conflicted heroine Piper's overly earnest sister-in-law Neri, all breastmilk and wraps and attachment parenting, has taken her on a wilderness retreat. The leader has invited them to shoot an arrow at a target, taking aim and releasing something that's been holding them back. Neri steps forward, wild-eyed, and hoists the bow. "I don't feel like a mom!" she cries. "Just me, with a baby." And she lets the arrow rip.

This is *exactly* how I feel. No better, no worse. No more nurturing just because I now have someone to nurture. Same strengths, same weaknesses; same sense of humor, same personality flaws; same me. With babies.

I think a lot about our cultural narrative of motherhood, of good mothers and bad, and of what it means to be someone's mother at all. Our conversations tend to circle around heroism or sacrifice, or both. Think of the headlines praising the mother who lifts a car off her kid, lent superhuman strength by love. Of the paeans to cancer-stricken pregnant women who go without treatment to save their fetuses, wasting away as the babies grow. Marmee from *Little Women*, loving and sorrowful, a Madonna in a dun-colored twice-mended dress. From the outside, my mother's obsession with me looked like devoted motherhood, universally laudable. As long as you didn't look too close.

What I really want is to be unremarkable. I want my children to take me more or less for granted, one more connection in a life full of them, one resource among a thousand available to them. The more important I am to them, I can't help thinking, the more I have the power to hurt them. The worse my legacy will be. A friend who lost her mother in her twenties still spends her limited vacation days, decades later, traveling to "Motherless Daughters" retreats. I don't want my kids to be so entwined with me that my inevitable loss defines them so much. I don't want to be their story the way that Warren was mine.

✦ ✦ ✦

When Rachel was four months old, we took her to meet my mother. She had met her over FaceTime, the phone wielded by her doctor, who inexplicably made weekly house calls to his difficult patient. Rachel examined the strip of my mother's hairline and the top of her glasses—the only part of her visible—with great interest, gurgling, cooing, and generally playing the part of the beloved grandchild to perfection. This was the relationship I had wanted—my loving mother mirroring my adoration for my baby girl, the Movie Moment—but the trap door of her mental state intervened. She was besotted, but not too besotted to resist breaking into shouts of recrimination and anger when I said it was time for Rachel to eat, as the doctor's worried face bobbed back into view and he ended the call.

Ever since I'd left for college, my mother had supplemented the rent with roommates in the two extra bedrooms, the maid's room shoehorned into the crook of the kitchen's L barely big enough for a twin bed and a custom hanging system where hangers hung parallel to the wall to save space. It was occupied by a graduate student named May, so shy she communicated only by notes left on the front hall table. The roommate currently in my old bedroom was, unusually, American, a veteran named Eric with a small rescue dog and five children with two different ex-wives. He made jokes I didn't care for about duct-taping my mom's mouth when she got too cranky. He'd bragged to me over email about how much he was helping her, which struck me as strange—she had Medicaid-paid aides coming in eight hours a day, seven days a week—but he was clearly eccentric and she was happy, and so for a while I let it be. They were two lonely older people keeping each other company; what could be more natural?

She wanted us to come to the apartment. I vetoed that quick-like. She bristled, but I pointed out that my memories of months-long stints of childhood bronchitis were still fresh, and the clouds of yellow smoke in her apartment were a no-go for a tiny infant. I was unreasonable, she said. Overemotional and irrational. But magnanimously she finally agreed, and we settled on brunch at her neighborhood diner, the kind of place where you order eggs by the number and where a refrigerator case full of cheesecake and improbably high coconut meringue cake rotates sedately by the counter.

They came in together, my mother on Eric's arm. My first thought when I saw him was an arch *two ex-wives, oh REALLY*, but had you seen the studded duster layered over a Broadway musical T-shirt, the gleaming bald head, and the piercings up

and down his wrinkled ears, I suspect you'd forgive me. He was
fussing over my mother like a cartoon nursemaid, and when
she spotted Rachel sitting in my lap, swatting at a salt shaker,
she burst into tears. Eric helped her onto the bench seat and
greeted us all effusively; we allowed, guardedly, that it was nice
to meet him. I put Rachel into my mother's arms. She gathered
her against her stained white sweatshirt and wrapped her hands
around Rachel's tiny body. For one moment, I allowed myself
the image: my mother meeting her first grandchild, suffused
with love, perfect and pure and not yet slashed through with fury
and guilt. Tears coursed down her cheeks, and she let out a half
moan, half ecstatic yawp; for a Jewish woman of her generation,
the introduction of the grandchild was a moment you longed for
from the instant your own children cleared the cervix. Gamely,
Rachel peered into her face, registered her tears, then whipped
her head around and looked at us forlornly. I could smell the
Marlboros from across the table.

"I brought her a cupcake!" said my mother. "It's her four-
month birthday." (It wasn't.)

"That's very sweet of you, Mom, thanks," I said, and Eric
pulled a boxed cupcake and a candle out of a shopping bag. Her
grip was loose, and I saw Rachel slipping a half-centimeter at a
time toward the tiled floor. "Let me hold her, OK?"

"No, it's *my* turn! You took four *months* to bring my grandchild to me—"

"Judith, *sha, sha*," Eric scolded, flapping his hands at her.
"The baby's mother wants to hold her, give her back." *Oh
honey*, I thought. *Using her first name and telling her no? They'll
never find your body.* But amazingly, she let me take Rachel back
without another word and I felt a wash of gratitude toward
this bizarre character to whom my mother seemed to listen.

Arie set up the cupcake and we blew out the candle on Rachel's behalf, much to her delight; my mother and Eric applauded her giggles. The hovering waiter took our orders and brought pancakes and eggs, chunky white mugs of coffee.

"She's *cold*, you didn't even *dress* her enough. Here, I'll fix it," my mother snapped, and started to take off her own sweatshirt. I caught an expanse of skin and the pilled fabric of an old bra. She was wearing nothing under it. "*No!*" Eric and I barked together, and he pulled her shirt down for her. "I was going to give it to her as a blanket," she said, injured. Arie caught my eye and shook his head slightly. *We just have to get through this hour*, he telegraphed. My mother was playing peekaboo with a skeptical and perfectly warm Rachel, blissfully unaware.

She peered over her bifocals into Rachel's tiny face, and screwed up her mouth. "She doesn't look like you," she said to Arie, sniffing. "Are you sure she's yours?" Arie smiled politely, his mouth tight. Eric swatted her arm and rolled his eyes at me. The presence of this flamboyant child-man there with us was a blessing in disguise. It absolved me from having to shush her. I was no longer concerned that Eric was going to murder her in her sleep for her Social Security checks. They were two peas in a dysfunctional, faux-Yiddish-accented pod, and I was relieved to have her eyes on someone else for a little while.

I emptied half-and-halfs into a series of coffee refills and counted the minutes until we could leave. The force of her love—and the embarrassment of her shrill harassment of the waiters and intermittent yelling—put my every nerve on edge. I had known this wouldn't be a perfect, pastoral scene of grandmother meeting granddaughter, but I had also not anticipated a close call with public nudity. You could say this for my mother: she'd surprise you every time.

She sat the rest of the meal with her head cocked to the side, her eyes damp and focused on Rachel's curious little face. When we stood up to leave, I handed the baby to my mother for a final hug, standing close enough to grab her if she fell. She kissed the top of Rachel's head and gave her back. "She's just as beautiful as you were, Miss Mouse," she said shakily, and I felt my eyes prickle with tears. We buckled Rachel back into the car seat and fled, leaving Eric to escort her home.

I saw my mother's inability to be a functional grandparent much earlier than I was able to understand her inability to be a parent. And man, I was not my best self when that happened. I felt betrayed by the unfairness of it all over again, and then excoriated myself for the self-pity. When my dear friend Gabriela got pregnant, I thought about her often-traveling airline pilot husband and offered to come over when the baby was born and hold it while she napped, to run errands, clean the bathroom—all the things we had not had someone there to do in a new city with a new baby. "Oh," she said matter-of-factly, "that's so sweet! But Mom is coming up for the first few months, so she'll be there every day."

I wanted only the best for my friend, and I was relieved she wouldn't be left alone with a newborn—but also, oh, I fumed. I fucking seethed. Another friend's mother, recently released from prison, left the halfway house and stayed in her guest room, babysitting for my friend's young sons so she and her husband could go out to dinner in clothes unstained with spit-up. Snakes of envy twisted in my stomach. "She's a literal *felon*, she literally can't take the kids to the playground because of her *ankle monitor*, but I'm still jealous," I raged to Arie. "Because Anne can trust her mother alone with her kids, and

I can't." I hated how I sounded, so outraged and self-pitying, but I couldn't help myself.

Of course these people I envied so bitterly had their own troubles. It's the worst and oldest cliché that you never really know what's going on in someone's home, and that the most adorable, sickeningly perfect family photo can obscure a family hellscape. I learned from my mother that people can hide a lot more than a concealer-spackled bruise or a recycling bin full of bottles. I learned that if you're born outside a hospital, you never need a birth certificate. I learned that you can get a passport with your childhood immunization records and your school transcript and a few other pieces of hastily cobbled together ID. I learned that you can live in the same house with someone who is lying to you about not only who she is, but about who you are, *and you will never know*.

She created a whole fake world for me, soup to nuts. In her world, my Vietnam vet father was my mother's husband, was named Warren Steven Livingston, and had died innocently in a tragic car crash. She had lived chastely ever since, focused only on being a mother. In her world we subsisted on her savings. Her accommodating young mini-me got good grades and had perfect manners. And it was all completely fake. This was less gaslighting than window dressing; I was the smallest doll on her stage, the youngest plot device in her story. All the while, she was a) still married, b) sleeping with another woman's husband, and c) standing outside the bathroom shrieking while the mini-me held her ground inside.

I play a little game with myself. When I've known someone for a while, long enough to trust them, I think: What part of this story could be fake? What have I actually seen happen, what documentation has actually crossed my eyes, what part of this could be untrue? Does she really live in that house? Is he really married? Is that really her name? You can make just about anything sound fictional just by thinking through what it would really take to fool you.

My kids are still too young to know a lie from a truth. Stalwart in his disdain for dishonesty, my husband won't tell them even the tiny lies of childhood; when Rachel falls, he asks her if "placebo magic" will help, and then does a complicated dap that gets a smile back on her face. Left to my own parental devices I'd probably punt on some of these, but I do wonder what I *should* tell them about their raging, absent grandmother, about their long-dead grandfather. What's the right cautionary tale when they come home smelling like breath mints, guilty over half a stolen beer? Their booze-sodden great-grandmother prostrate on the living room floor? Their young, handsome grandfather making a half-turn in the air before hitting the pavement with a crack? Their twenty-something mother starting stupid fights with friends, waking up headachy and shaky and not remembering to whom she needs to apologize?

How long can I just keep my mouth shut?

CHAPTER 12

A Room Full of Men

I left for New York in the middle of a monsoon, my leaking rain boots hastily mended with Minion-printed duct tape. An inauspicious beginning, I thought, clomping grimly up the steps of the bus with my overstuffed bag thumping against my knees. I was still breastfeeding four-month-old Rachel and I pumped in the bus bathroom, praying no one would need the single reeking toilet.

I was light-headed with anticipation. Aside from my mother, whose memory of him was dim, I had never looked another human being in the face who had known Warren. His high school classmates had invited me to his fiftieth reunion. These men had known Warren *as* Warren, not as the blank, father-shaped cipher in my own mind.

The rain was heavy and the bus was late. At Port Authority, I pumped again in the restroom and changed into my cocktail dress and heels, hopping to keep my feet off the filthy floor in the process. The traitorous boots had sprung more leaks between DC and New York; I slung them victoriously into a trash bin and started speed-walking. There was no time to drop off my stuff at Yumi's, where I was staying the night. It wasn't the polished Audrey Hepburn entrance I'd planned, but neither, thankfully, was it Lucille Ball stuffing chocolates into her cleavage.

The opening ceremony of the reunion was in the beautiful, old-money school chapel on the Upper West Side. I sat in the back goggling at the men around me, from cane-wielding elder statesmen to gangly frat boys. It didn't look at all like my all-women's college reunions. No small children weaving through the crowd; no shrieks of delighted recognition; no chanting school songs in Greek, which, fair enough.

Mostly I was fascinated to see what this kind of money looked like. A year at Collegiate, even for a kindergartner, cost more than an undergraduate's year at Harvard. Who were these men whose families could afford this kind of education, and who had they been?

They were white, no surprise there. They were amiable. I'd kind of been expecting titans of industry, wheeling, dealing, and sweet-talking each other, or barking orders at stoic spouses. Nope. No fancy suits, no heads-together networking. These were beaming, sweet-faced middle-aged men vigorously shaking hands, delighted to meet each other again after so many years, to see the well-remembered younger faces shining out from under the wrinkles and progressive lenses.

Wealth hung more obviously on the younger alumni. They were dressed nicely if casually, jeans and sports jackets, heads in their phones, accompanied by glossy-haired young women from Chapin and Spence and Brearley. You could never have mistaken me and my scruffy high school friends for them. They were steeped in cheerful carelessness, interested in the proceedings in an affable, offhanded kind of way. A party was being thrown for them, like parties had always been thrown for them; nothing new to see here.

The speeches began, jovial and earnest. I couldn't pay attention. My head swiveled around on my shoulders. *He should* be *here*, I thought. He should be wearing a diffident suit, clapping his friends on the shoulder, joking about a bum knee or a memory that wasn't what it used to be. He should be delighted to see his old bandmates and friends. He should still be moving through the world, a little creakier than he'd been. I squared my shoulders and stared upward, an old trick to stop tears from hitting my cheeks.

When the ceremony ended, the roar of conversation rose quickly. I escaped out the rear. Back in the school for the cocktail reception, I stalled out, skulking like a creeper past the chipper welcomers and name tag hander-outers. Too nervous to join the reception, I tip-tapped furtively up the main stairs of the Upper School. There's something about visiting a school as an adult that makes you feel like you're still beholden to all the rules and the punishments, like they might still catch you; you might feel a security guard's heavy hand on your shoulder, or find yourself squeezing into a too-small desk for detention. But no one was there. The stone steps were worn down in the middle from decades of careless teenage feet, and the hallways smelled surprisingly familiar: chalk, the tang of marker, sweat.

It was an electrifying sensation. He had walked in these hallways. He had run down them late to class, slammed a locker door, shoulder-checked classmates, hid the sour breath of hangovers. I had never before stood in a room where I knew Warren had been. I felt sure I could smell him—hearty and jocular, the musky smell of young sweat. I closed my eyes and tried to hear his ghost, thinking of his classmate's story of him standing outside the school belting out "Gee, Officer Krupke" (a favorite of my own) "with somewhat indifferent success but great enthusiasm." Warren sounded like a party. In high school I would have been afraid of him, not cool enough to talk to him, but in my early twenties we would have been drinking buddies.

In the basement, long, winding corridors spiked off the gym. A black-painted room marked "Senior Lounge" boasted low-slung couches, a gaming system, and a Coke machine. Did students really hang out in a school-provided lounge? At my own 90s-era high school, taking advantage of any official space would have been relentlessly uncool. Maybe the wealthy kids of the 60s saw a space like this as an unremarkable birthright, one more hand provided to cast down the red carpet and chill the drink.

This was, I thought, the kind of shadow life I might have lived had I been born where I was born, only thirty years earlier and with piles of money.

I made a full circuit, then another. This was stupid. *I* was being stupid. I rolled my shoulders, breathed deep, and walked into the cocktail hour. It was loud and already rowdy, a thousand cheerful decibels of male excitement. Ties had been loosened and jackets unbuttoned, faces were flushed. I was one of only a few women there, but no one seemed to be looking for me. I found a bar line to stand in and stood in it, gratefully.

Peeling the label from my beer, I steeled myself and inched around the room, peering at the name tags of all the men who looked to be around the right age. A white-haired elder statesman–looking type materialized out of the crowd, our eyes met, and he smiled, politely but vaguely, like you might smile at someone you just missed knocking into in a hallway. I sidled up and peered at his name tag. Bingo. The two men talking to him turned and smiled expectantly.

"*Hglrph*," I said indistinctly. "*Hrmph!*" I cleared my throat. "Paul. Hello. I'm Liz Scheier. Warren's daughter. Warren Luther?" *STOP TALKING*, I instructed myself.

He broke into a wide, guileless smile. "*Liz!* Oh my goodness. Look at you. Well. It certainly *is* you." I grinned, precariously, and pawed the ground like a talking horse at a fair. He introduced me to a few men around me, whose names I forgot the moment they were said, and I ducked my head, still grinning. The inside of my head was white, like a blinding flash had gone off. Someone had looked at me and seen Warren. Someone had seen *Warren*, and then had seen *me*, and had found a connection between us to be plausible. I was lit up from the inside. I was aflame. My empty man-shape of a father had been somewhere, had walked somewhere, had spoken to other human beings; he had touched things. He was in the background of someone's pictures. He had sweated on a bench, shed dandruff on a desk, missed the urinal when shaking off, jerked off in a stall, spat on the sidewalk outside. His physical body had touched their physical bodies, had touched the stone and wood and cement of this school. He had been *real*. He was gone but he had been *real*. I was on the tremulous verge of tears, and stepped hard on my toe with the other heel to stop them.

They invited me to their post-reunion dinner, we made small talk, and I politely excused myself, not wanting to intrude on their conversation by having a public nervous breakdown. I would like to say that I spent the rest of the cocktail hour familiarizing myself with the school, or introducing myself to people, or any other useful and productive occupation. I did not. I spent it hiding in the bathroom.

They'd reserved a private room at a French restaurant near the school, and my sense of not belonging reared up when I realized I didn't know the name on the reservation: "It's a reunion!" I tried. "Of . . . mostly men? Older men?" The maître d' took pity on me and led me down a dark, red-wallpapered hallway hung with framed hunting sketches. Old-school masculinity stretched to its extreme like Silly Putty, a cliché of itself.

The private back room was half-filled with sixtysomething men, chatting and laughing, Paul among them. He jumped to his feet and hurried over. "Gentlemen!" he said to the room. "This is Warren's daughter." They erupted into *hello*s and shoulder pats and handshakes, beaming; I wondered if this was what it was like to be presented to old friends by a proud father, and tried to look civilized and worthy. A waiter handed me a glass the size of a small globe, and I took a mouthful of wine and held it, relying on the bite of tannins to keep me from saying anything ridiculous. Men strode over to me or sidled over one at a time, reminiscing about Warren. This party, that concert, a host of football games. *My dad was a* jock, I thought, wonderingly.

As we finished our giant portions of steak—stricken with an anxious nausea so deep I didn't dare stand up, I ate very little—Robert stood in his official capacity as the class alumni representative and welcomed the group. He spoke briefly and introduced the guests. I tried not to look crazed as I smiled. I was hyperaware of being somewhere I only nominally belonged.

Robert was roundly catcalled, and the group erupted into brief barks of laughter over happy memories. An early-twenties son who was clearly humoring his father by showing up tipped back in his chair with a bored expression, swinging his legs. I hated him for finding the whole thing burdensome, when for me it was so shocking and miraculous to even be in this company. There was a pall over the room. There had been only thirty or so students in his class. Out of those thirty, two others had committed suicide—Warren hadn't even been the youngest—and one had lost both a younger brother and a son to suicide, all drinking-related. I looked around at them all. Half of them sat with virtuous glasses of seltzer in their hands.

I had known kids from those private schools; I went to Hebrew school with them. I had envied them. They had parents, usually two, who were presentable in public. They clattered through the hallways in slick winter jackets clacking with lift tickets, vacationed in places I couldn't pronounce, looked forward to uncomplicated futures. Or that's what I'd thought. These men must once have looked just as put-together, just as untouchable. But their homes had been falling apart, and alcohol had—literally—decimated their ranks.

This was nothing to envy. It's a greeting-card sentiment, but their wealth hadn't protected them. Smoothed the corners, maybe, and covered a few months of rehab here and there, but also paid for those gallons of 7 and 7s and those parties.

I made it to my feet, hugged them all, promised to keep in touch, and showed one more round of pictures of the infant Rachel on demand. I threw myself into a cab and drew my knees into my chest for the silent ride downtown. I let myself into Yumi's empty apartment, making it to the toilet just in time to throw up my guts.

CHAPTER 13

The Apple and the Tree

March was always a shit month for my mother. Every year, she emerged from winter grimmer than she entered it. As an adult I played hooky from Passover, remembering the tight-lipped silence as she stabbed moodily at pans of matzah brei and swept crumbs out of cabinets into a wooden spoon with a purple feather rescued from a discarded boa, simmering with barely repressed sadness. In that first apartment on First Avenue, she took the "let all who are hungry come and eat" line literally, inviting anyone from a nearby nursing home who didn't have another seder to go to. She set up folding tables down the foyer into the living room, draping them with hand-embroidered and ironed linens, and presided at the head with half the guests nodding sleepily in their wheelchairs.

Most of the guests had never seen a woman run a seder before. Older women beamed at her when their husbands weren't looking, signaling a genteel *attagirl* with their whole bodies. My buffoon of a cousin—a man I only saw once a year, if that—signaled his displeasure by jumping on all the good lines. "NEXT YEAR IN MIAMI BEACH!" he'd boom, and "Let my people go *to bed*, haven't we about wrapped up here, Judith?" She'd glare at him over her bifocals and he'd settle down, crestfallen, until his next opportunity to interrupt.

During those brief and damp New York springs I often came upon her weeping, standing by the floor-to-ceiling bookshelves in the living room, paging through ancient Book of the Month Club editions of dull-looking novels. I didn't know why spring got her down so badly until I was old enough to understand the tiny candle flickering for a night and a day in its delicate glass jar.

My maternal grandmother was forty-four when she died. In a picture taken a few months before her death, Ruth is dancing with my uncle Phil at his bar mitzvah. She weighs barely sixty pounds, and her bright, mournful eyes shine above cheekbones slender and sharp as scalpels. She didn't know she was dying, or if she did, it was only because she'd guessed. The family doctor had admonished my mother to keep the severity of Ruth's illness—a quick-spreading cancer in her colon—from her. *If she knew how sick she was it could discourage her*, he said. *It could make things worse.*

And so they told her, against all immediate and obvious evidence, that she was getting better.

When Ruth died, my mother—a freshman at Barnard—went back to the Far Rockaway house to find it sold, furnishings and belongings along with the bricks and glass. Her textbooks, her photographs, her furniture—all of it now belonged to someone else. Ruth's husband, Lou—a Catskills Borscht Belt comedian (think Mrs. Maisel lampooning her father, or the scenes at Kellerman's in *Dirty Dancing*)—had taken my teenage uncle Phil on the road, yanking him out of middle school. He never went back.

I've seen the house where she grew up (or, well, where she says she did). It's a perfectly ordinary house on a street full of houses just like it, near the beach in Belle Harbor, Queens, New York City. She has never told me details of her childhood, but she makes it seem like American Family Paradise: mother, father, two children, big stick-fetching dogs, cousins next door. Our own home, by contrast, was marked by what it didn't contain. She grieved not for my father, but for the fact that he wasn't there; she mourned my lack of family and the distance of my grown-up-with-kids-of-their-own cousins.

Shortly before Ruth died, she sent my mother a letter on hospital stationery. The handwriting is cramped and tense, rounded like copperplate. "Dearest," she says, "I want to tell you a story and writing it so I shouldn't leave anything out + I may get weepy if I talk about it. I will try to be very clinical about it—altho there is no point or moral to it but that we can understand each other better. There are many things that I shall say, that I have never revealed before."

It goes on to tell the story of the men she dated before my mother's father, whom she married a year to the day before my mother was born. Their marriage was an unhappy one. Herb traveled often for work, and he spoke unkindly to her when he was home, and went out with other women when he wasn't. They split before their second anniversary, and Ruth moved with my infant mother to live with my great-grandparents. The war with Germany was just starting. She planted a victory garden— well, hired someone to plant a victory garden—and played with my toddler mother when she felt well enough. Barely any time passed before she met her second husband, and she clearly thought herself lucky, as she finishes the letter this way:

"But please believe me when I say that Daddy + I both love you so much as you actually brought us together. I don't even think that Daddy would have noticed me if it weren't for you because I am so nondescript + uninteresting—just like a plough horse.

Mom"

Well.

This is astonishing to me. Ruth wrote this letter when she was, (probably) unbeknownst to her, near death. The letter is undated, but my mother couldn't have been older than 18. What would lead someone to write this to a young woman? Was it a coy invitation—*tell me it's not true, tell me I'm pretty*? Who *says* something like this? And why?

The copy is missing the page in which Lou and Ruth met and fell in love. This could be an accident, but the page could have contained a memory too painful in retrospect for my mother to pass along. I have only Ruth's final, miserable self-assessment by which to judge. If I look at this letter and wonder what kind of man is obsessed enough with a small girl that he will marry her mother for access to her, I want to believe that's my own skepticism, my own modern sensibility. My paranoia, built of a childhood in which my mother never allowed me to be alone in a room with a man, and almost never let me out of her sight at all, even to go to school. Most likely, that missing page is just an innocent play-by-play of their meeting. Or the retelling is misdirection, Ruth's skewed attempt to tell her daughter how much she loves her: Look, darling, people have changed their lives for you. The world revolves around you. I will make it yours.

In the same pile of papers, I found a stack of wartime letters Ruth wrote to her estranged husband, my biological grandfather. Her tone shifting between airy, patriotic, and mopey, she blames and forgives him by turns, and I start to think that perhaps this is the trauma the books about borderline personality disorder talk about—my mother's abandonment by her first father. It gave me some understanding of the formula she was working from. The absent father, the constrained finances. The mother and her young daughter, abandoned. The two of them against the world. The girl responsible for her mother's happiness, the pivot around which the world revolved.

But they are gone and they were liars, all of them. There is no way to know for sure.

✦ ✦ ✦

In October 2015, Mom had called me to ask if I could help her with rent. I was burned out. My breakup was still fresh, I had just moved into a new, more expensive apartment, my kidney transplant was a week away, and I was still gun-shy from many years of paying her substantial bills and helping out with errands only to be screamed at for not doing enough. I said no, I was about to go on medical leave and my job wasn't going well, it wasn't the right time. She rushed to say no problem, no, forget it, it would all work out.

That was the month she stopped paying her rent again.

Adult Protective Services called a year and a half later, after the wedding and the move to DC and the first baby. I answered a call on the way to daycare, huffing and puffing in the searing DC heat. It was an unknown number, with a caseworker on the other end, asking if I knew that my mother was being evicted that week, and that I was named in the lawsuit—a lawsuit that had already gone to court several times and been adjourned. The summons for which had arrived, every time, addressed to me at my mother's apartment, "nailed and mailed" to the door of a place where I hadn't lived in decades.

I sat down on a bench outside the daycare building and lowered my sweating forehead between my knees. I had a non-lawyer's fear of brushing up against the legal system. We had just bought a house and had cast in our lot with a city where most good jobs were government, which meant background checks, which meant a clean record, which meant *don't get sued*. I had been on the lease all along, ever since we'd moved in in 1985. I was six years old. My mother had paid the previous tenant $20,000 in cash to transfer the lease; there were whispers of the building going co-op, meaning she'd have first dibs on buying the apartment. It never did. A three-bedroom, three-bathroom half a block from Central Park, it was then on the southern end of Morningside Heights—not the most attractive of neighborhoods—but by the time this eviction notice arrived, she was paying a rent-stabilized $2,000 a month on a $7,000 market-rate apartment. The landlord had plenty of reason to want her out.

I don't know what happened in October. Maybe her narrow margin of cash slimmed down so that she just couldn't write the check. Maybe she misplaced the cash, or maybe one of her aides stole it. I still have no idea where the cash her roommates were giving her went. There were other setbacks. When Eric-the-weird-roommate abruptly lost his job in the Garment District, he stopped paying rent. Subdued, he assured me over email that he was applying for Social Security, and suggested that the "help" he was providing her might somehow suffice as payment. I shut that down quickly.

She finally kicked him out, flailing and raging, with the help of the police, half a year in the hole. Her other roommate, May, who was reporting a New Jersey address to avoid paying New York City taxes, would not sign a form confirming that she lived there and was helping with rent. With no proof that she was making any attempt at all to make the payments, all city programs that provide short-term assistance turned her down.

She'd broken her nearly perfect twenty-five-year rent payment record, and she never wrote another check.

Every two years I'd signed that lease along with her. Looking back, I don't know why. Her argument was that it was a gift to me, that one day I would move into the apartment and take over the stabilized rent. I joked about it being my inheritance. For those of you not from New York, this is not as crazy as it sounds. Plenty of people do it. A summer camp friend had moved herself and her new husband into her childhood apartment, and her mother segmented off a bedroom and mini-kitchen for herself. A child came, then another, and still they all stayed. That lease kept them all housed in a city that got more absurdly expensive by the day. It would have been an incredible deal, but I couldn't imagine doing it. The thought of living in that apartment—hanging my work clothes in the same closets where I had hidden squashed in the back as she raged, or showering in the bathroom where I tremblingly unlocked the door while she stood outside holding the whimpering dog—made my stomach turn. I could paint the walls, cover the nicotine-yellowed paint. I could switch out the furniture, change the locks, purge the smell of smoke. But the bones would always be there.

She had pulled a lot of nearly unbelievable shit in her time.

But none of it had put me in harm's way—from an outside source, at least. Certain there had to be something wrong with the caseworker's story, I called my mother from home, the air conditioner blasting. DC summers are no fucking joke. I was already pregnant again, and I got home every day with a baby-shaped circle of sweat on my dress where I carried Rachel in her wrap, perched above the bump of her brother.

She sounded, as ever, delighted to hear from me. "Well *hi*, you! How is my beautiful granddaughter? You should call back later when Dr. Anand is here, we can do that face thing, you know, the video—"

"Mom," I interrupted. "Hang on. Did you get an eviction notice from the landlord?"

A beat. "Who told you that?"

Up until that moment, I had hoped it was a mistake. Messily dated paperwork from the last time the landlord had tried to evict her, maybe, or a well-meaning but mistaken neighbor. *It can't be possible*, I thought, *that my own mother wouldn't tell me she'd gotten me sued.*

"That doesn't matter. Mom, my name is on that lawsuit. I'm going to need a lawyer. If this had gone to judgment, we wouldn't have been able to get the mortgage. What did you—"

She laughed abrasively, a familiar, unpleasant bark of a sound that conveyed neither hilarity nor joy, but a warning to shut my mouth. "Oh *Elizabeth*, you don't know *anything*. That's not *true*, none of that is true. I'm handling it, and it's none of your business."

"Handling it how? If you haven't paid rent in a year, you owe almost $25,000. Where are you planning on—"

"I'm not listening to this! I don't have to listen to *any* of this. I am the parent and you are the child and my finances are none of your business. Stop *hassling* me, Elizabeth. I'm not *well*, you can't *do* this."

"But it's not just *your* finances! My name is on there too—"
And she hung up.

I realized my mouth was open, and I shut it with a snap. I had expected a refutation, or perhaps a defensive insistence that it was my fault for not giving her rent money more than a year ago. I had not imagined that she would completely deny that it was happening at all.

This was the sitcom version of my mother, the Cantankerous Jewish Matriarch character she'd put on for so many years, teasing and blustering, trying to get a laugh out of people. But it seemed that the caricature was now real. Dementia? Worsening mental illness? Just general age-related crankiness? Was it shame? Had she convinced herself she could somehow just talk her way out of this?

No way to know. But inside, I felt the fraying hemp of the last ropes tying me to her creak to their breaking point. I have forgiven my mother for a lot of things over the years. Some in light of her illness, and some because it's just exhausting to be that angry for that long and I ran out of energy to keep it up. But this was something new. I could not forgive the yearlong silence, the deliberate hiding of the lawsuit with my name on it. She had gone to court multiple times, with the city-provided attorney, and every time, she'd sat silently when the judge asked who was there representing me. Just the fact of the lawsuit made us ineligible for insurance; had there been a judgment, it would have curtailed my DC career forever. I could have been on the hook for the five figures in rent she hadn't told me she'd stopped paying. We had just bought a house, and the mortgage—my first—hung over my head.

I stopped returning her calls. I had never picked up every one—during her worst manic phases she would call ten or fifteen times a day—but my pick-ups petered out and one day I just stopped. For almost a year, she continued calling every Friday night to wish us a good Shabbos and other times as she thought of it, never once mentioning that I hadn't returned her last call, or any of her calls. I don't know if she remembered that I hadn't.

I did what women have always done; I cut off the risk to my children. This reminder of how dangerous she could be made me quail when I thought of them caught up in her vortex. I did for them what I had never been able, in forty years, to do for myself—admit that taking responsibility for insanity only spreads the insanity around.

I finally called from the hospital, my voice deep and heavy with exhaustion, to tell her that I had had a son. We had not spoken in almost a year. She heard the name, remembered enough to note that his middle name was my father's, and then said, with high-pitched incredulity, "Elizabeth—I feel like I haven't spoken to you in a while. Are you *angry* with me?"

I looked at David Warren, his smushy little red face screwed up in sleep against Arie's chest. I had shifted while speaking, and the swollen, traumatized skin around my vagina screamed. I just couldn't do it. "We can talk about that another time," I said, and hung up.

We never did. I knew that bringing it up would lead only to one of her two poles, the fury or the grief. I would hear how she had done nothing wrong, how I was wrong, how I wasn't named in the suit, how the case had never gone to court, how there was no case at all, how courts as a concept didn't even exist, and what was wrong with me; or I would hear that yes, she was a terrible parent, she was the worst parent, she had been so terrible to me when I was a child. She was the living embodiment of Anne Lamott's description of Radio KFKD, Radio K-Fucked, which streamed an endless patter of insults into one ear and a river of relentless self-aggrandizement into the other; she was the piece of shit around which the world revolved. When the mother of an elementary school friend of mine, with whom she had been friendly, died of lung cancer, she told me wistfully that my friend's teenage sister had then taken up smoking because the smell of cigarettes reminded her of her mother. "You would never love me that much," she said, half-joking. She wanted to prod me into a protestation of filial love, but she also kind of meant it. If in order to show your love for your mother you had to start smoking the poison that killed her; light up, kid.

It took me almost forty years, and the experience of being an adult in a house full of small children, to understand what I had not seen then. Yes, she could be a monster. Yes, her rage and her violence were terrifying. But more than that, I had grown up in a house with no competent adults in it. We lacked supervision. We rattled around that apartment like two children, one oblivious and one overgrown, who'd buried the babysitter in the back garden and had no idea what to do next. Neither of us had any idea how to exist in the world of normal people.

I called the kind but overworked APS caseworker back many times over that next year, trying to get more of the story, as she struggled to put the pieces together herself. My mother had grown increasingly secretive and refused to tell her when the hearings were happening. Her aide started calling me furtively from other rooms, hanging up midsentence when she approached, with the dates she was supposed to go down to the courthouse. I got the name of the guardian ad litem, who as far as we could tell had never shown up for a hearing, and who never returned my voice mails. I raged futilely for months until the caseworker received a front-door photo series the GAL had logged with the court, time-stamped on a series of days that he'd gone to her apartment; she had repeatedly refused to let him in.

I got my own lawyer. He wrote a series of increasingly irate documents to the court pointing out that it can hardly have escaped the landlord's notice—given that there was a twenty-four-hour doorman—that I hadn't been inside the building in a year, and hadn't lived there in more than a decade. For the next year, I waited and cursed and paced and waited. And wrote checks. It took eight thousand dollars and ten excruciating months, but the landlord ultimately agreed to remove me from the lease in exchange for a signed statement that I was relinquishing my rights to the apartment. A wise move on their part. I could have passed that lease along to my own children, tying that prime apartment up in rent stabilization laws for another century.

In the meantime, APS filed twice to appoint her a personal guardian. Those court dates were added to the dozen eviction hearings, each of which ended with sympathetic judges giving her more time. The guardianships were denied. On the one hand, I couldn't argue with the judges' reluctance. It is no small thing to take away someone's agency and allow someone else control over their life. It shouldn't be easy to do that. But there is such a vast gap between the moment in time when a person starts to make decisions that are not just dubious but actively harmful, and the time when a court is willing to step in. Legally, she was still in bad decision territory, not catastrophe. She was crazy, everyone agreed. No question. Just not crazy enough.

So APS changed tacks, and petitioned for a financial guardian. By that time, she hadn't paid rent in two years, and the court agreed that this probably indicated a small issue with her ability to manage her finances. A city agency was appointed, and another well-intentioned but overworked caseworker called to ask, cheerily, when my mother could move in with me; she sounded a bit taken aback when I laughed. "You'll understand better the more you get to know her," I said grimly, and within a week, she agreed that there was no way in hell I was letting my mother near my kids. "She's not like . . . what I thought she was like," she said carefully. Which probably meant my mother had called her a cunt.

Here's what I learned over the course of those two years when she dragged around in that apartment like the last woman on earth. If you're an educated-sounding white lady with a reliable phone line and a persistent attitude, the social safety net is much more like a feather bed. Seven days a week, eight hours a day, she was attended by a series of pragmatic, caring home health-care aides sent by the city to do her laundry and her shopping and make sure she ate. The scatterbrained but determined social worker at Adult Protective Services called me weekly, trying everything—city grants, court appearances, roommate agreements—to keep her solvent and situated. When APS finally got a motion through, a guardian was appointed from a nonprofit agency to find her an alternate living situation. They were all dedicated and hardworking, schlepping out to her apartment week after week and following up off-hours.

These women—and they were all women—followed the same pattern. They started off confident, sure my mother was just like any other elderly client—eccentric, sure, cranky, definitely, but so funny! So charming!—and nothing they couldn't handle. All of them asked some initial pointed questions about why I wasn't there more, or helping more—I learned to recognize the sound of lips pursing over the phone—but over time, their calm turned to surprise, and then to incredulity, and finally to exasperation. Her stubbornness was unprecedented in their experience, and her inability to act in her own best interests confused and then alarmed them. I tried to keep the vindication out of my voice. I usually failed.

I did speak to her doctor, frequently. He was still making weekly house calls, a setup that initially gave me some comfort, which soon turned to confusion, and from there to mistrust. He showered me with praise and flattery, told my mother exactly what she wanted to hear, and, it turned out, cashed her Social Security checks for her. (Whether or not the money ever made it back to her was a mystery never solved.) On the rare occasions that I caught her in a calm or amenable mood and got her to agree to apply to an assisted living facility, he delayed returning the required forms—or returned them incorrectly, as many as six or seven different times in six or seven different ways—until the beds were no longer available. Add this to the list of things I didn't understand about the situation: Was he so eccentric or oblivious that he didn't understand he wasn't supposed to be involved in a patient's finances, was he just genuinely incapable of filling out a simple form? Or was he scheming to keep his adoring patient exactly where she was, under his care? There was no way to know what was really going on. Mom would hear nothing against him. He was telling her she was perfectly healthy and needed no help, and he showed up every week to listen to her stories and, I assume, billed those visits to Medicaid. As far as she was concerned, he was perfect. Far more perfect than her bullying nag of a daughter, who kept asking such unreasonable questions as "Why do you sound like you can't breathe?," "Why aren't you using your oxygen?," and "Where are you planning on living next month?" I seethed, but did nothing. At the least, there were some eyes on her. There was someone to find the body if it came to that.

When the eviction started to look like it was finally really happening, I booked movers to rescue the stuff that couldn't be replaced, under the guise of wanting it for our still-newish house and "for the grandchildren." She owned one item of value, an eighteenth-century hope chest inherited from her for-mer mother-in-law that had been owned by a mysterious Anna Pum, and which had been hilarious to me in childhood because it was inscribed with sober, hand-carved caps that looked like they spelled "Penis." There was also a giant painting done by her ex-husband, a copy of a painting of bamboo from the Met, that had lived on the dining room wall and for which I had some nostalgic affection. By then she was already more than $70,000 behind on the rent, a fact she didn't seem to know I knew. She was still convinced that she was going to get more roommates—she'd evicted Eric, and May had wisely absconded for less chaotic ground—and return to normal, and didn't seem to realize that she'd been blacklisted by the undergraduate housing boards that had yielded most of her tenants.

"I hate this woman! She comes in too late," she'd com-plained to me once over the phone.

"Well, she's an adult, Mom," I mustered. "You could get earplugs."

"I will *not*," she snapped. "I fixed *her*. I told her she's probably a trafficked sex slave." My heart sank. The young woman was Thai.

"*Mom*. You can't *say* that. It's racist."

"Don't you tell *me* about racism. I lived through Vietnam!"

But not, like, getting *napalmed*, I didn't say. I'm not sure waiting out the war with the Sunday edition of the *New York Times* and an impatient scowl is activism, exactly.

For years I had posted ads on Craigslist to help my mother find roommates. An under-market room with a private bathroom half a block from Central Park in a twenty-four-hour doorman building was a needle in a city full of hay, and responses flooded in. Even after the eviction order, she seemed sure that all I had to do was "call Craig"—the internet being a somewhat nebulous concept for her—and all her troubles would be over. I quailed at the thought of wasting anxious room seekers' time with a post for a home from which they too would likely be evicted soon enough, and put her off. My mother is not, as you may have gathered, the type who suffers being put off lightly.

She called the night before the movers were to arrive. Safe handling and an interstate move is not cheap, and the best quote we could get was as much as it had cost us to move our entire lives to DC—more than $3,000. "Did you call Craig?" she asked, puffing furiously. She had paid the super to drill a hole between her bedroom and the living room, and had stashed her oxygen tank in the living room and threaded the tubes through the hole so that she could smoke in bed with the mask pushed up jauntily onto her forehead without fear of blowing up the building.

"No," I said wearily. "There's an eviction order out. I can't—"

"Well then, I hope you don't think I'm doing you a *favor* if you won't even do this for me. When those movers come tomorrow, I'll just send them home!"

The last rope whined and snapped. We had already paid the nonrefundable fee. I'm not proud that a lot of my final straws in this situation were financial. She could wield all the ugly words she wanted; she could cause a metric ton of chaos. This I was used to. But Arie and I were working our asses off, and paying almost $4,000 a month in childcare (which was average for our neighborhood; what the actual fuck, America?) for the privilege of doing it. She was not going to waste my money, too.

Arie deftly relieved me of the phone. But the *grandchildren*, he said smoothly. Rachel and David shouldn't miss out on their mother's childhood toys and books because of this, should they? Wouldn't it be wonderful for the kids to grow up with these things? I consulted the ceiling for strength. This was why I'd married a lawyer.

Typing at high speed, I put up a quick mock ad and hit "publish." He glanced over and nodded; my truth-obsessed husband wouldn't lie even for a good cause. "Mrs. Scheier," he interrupted. "Mrs.—no, let me just finish, please. Please, let me finish. Elizabeth has put up the ad." A silence. "Yes, she can be very stubborn." A big smile in my direction. I threw a pillow at his head. "Sure. Sure. Absolutely. Have a good night." I had deleted the posting before he could even end the call. Our consciences were both assuaged by the letter of the law.

Listen, I've done worse.

Two days later, the chest arrived, lovingly wrapped. The painting went right on the wall in the dining room. Along with the furniture, she sent boxes and boxes of stuff she thought was important—Lord knows how she got a busy moving crew to stand around for this—and I went through it all while on maternity leave with David. There was no rhyme or reason to what she'd sent; one giant, full-to-the-brim box contained every page of my fifth-grade homework and piles of childish artwork. Far more important was the validation. These things had all really happened. I had not made up or misremembered them. It's easy and tempting to try to create a legend out of your own past, to exaggerate a splinter removal into wrenching Excalibur from the rock. We all tell ourselves who-we-are stories that are not precisely true. But more of my memories proved to be true than not.

There it all was, in merciless type. Here was the school application with the fake Social Security number. Here was an printed-out email to her brother, retained for posterity, proudly describing how she was so disappointed with a birthday gift—it was not, as she had requested, a framed photo of me—that she had thrown it back, literally, at my head. (I remembered that clearly—the light cardboard box hitting my forehead, my startled shout, the *thwap* as it hit the floor and we stared at each other, me horrified but not surprised, she righteous and rageful.) And more mysteries: here was stationery with a law firm name at the top including her own surname. Had she tried to start her own firm after leaving her job? Had she mocked it up to . . . what? Get an apartment? Get another job? What the *hell*?

The box smelled like Albolene and hair spray. Sure enough, the first item on top was a snaggle of hair, bursting out of an envelope from the Macy's sixth-floor hair salon. I remembered asking her for it on one of our trips there, fresh from some children's book where a child lovingly preserves a locket with her mother's hair in it. It was darker gold than I remembered, with no gray yet. A stranger's.

Below, in a pile, was a sheaf of mystery. Some of the mysteries were immediate: What is this numbered list of men's names? Whose is this phone number, scrawled on an index card? Who is in this photo? And some were just baffling. Why this newspaper? Why this magazine? What spoke to her about this article? Or was it just padding to keep the other items safe, and I was trying to make meaning out of makeshift bubble wrap?

It wasn't enough to account for the filing cabinet. I stacked everything neatly in a cardboard box and shoved it in a corner of the attic. *Someday*, I thought, *I'll find the rest.*

✦ ✦ ✦

A peppy court evaluator called, wanting to get the full picture of my mother's health. "Now let's talk stairs," she said. I heard pages flipping in the background.

"Stairs?"

"Stairs, yeah. Does your house have a lot? I understand she has some trouble walking."

I silently counted to ten. "I think there may have been a misunderstanding. I have young children, and my mother isn't allowed near them. She can't move into my house."

A pause. "She isn't allowed near them? Do you mind if I ask why?"

I chose my words carefully. "She's a violent woman who can't control her rages, and I'm not going to let her do to them what she did to me."

"I see." I heard scribbling. "Honestly, Ms. Scheier, I have a lot more interview questions here, but if I pass along to the judge that the defendant's daughter believes her to be a danger to her own grandchildren, I suspect he'll consider that a fairly clear picture of her situation."

"Say what you need to say," I said firmly. "But she's not coming here."

The landlord continued to serve eviction notices. Reasonably; as shitty as they'd sometimes been over the years, I couldn't argue with almost three years of unpaid rent. Every time she got one, she'd get her aide to wrestle her and her oxygen tank into a cab, go down to housing court, and get an emergency stay of eviction. Judges saw a tiny elderly woman in a ratty housedress breathing through a cannula and ordered stay after stay. On one memorable occasion in August she had an eviction hearing adjourned because, she claimed, it was too hot in the chilly air-conditioned courtroom and she couldn't breathe; she then marched her aide out of the courthouse and sat them down at an outdoor cafe . . . that the judge passed on the way to his own lunch. Things started to go downhill for her after that.

I was accustomed to being lied to. I had made my peace with verifying every statement that came out of her mouth. What took some getting used to was learning to piece together a story from a variety of sources, some of them overworked, some of them refracted through dementia. You know the old joke about the blind men feeling parts of an elephant and naming what they've found—the man holding the trunk thinks he has a garden hose, the one holding the tail proudly hoists his whip? The picture I put together was always informed by the last person I talked to, and constrained by what they remembered. The court evaluator could confirm that the Jackass Doctor had shown up at a hearing, but left too early to hear what he testified; the social worker thought the judge was annoyed

at her, but didn't know the outcome; the court docket listed
a verdict, but in muddled language even my lawyer husband
didn't understand; and my mother herself insisted everything
was fine, *fine*, and when was I bringing her grandchildren to
visit and renting her a new apartment?

She was wobbling somewhere between needing assistance
with the Activities of Daily Living—bathing, dressing, and
toileting—and just needing somewhere to lay her head at night.
Because her own sense of reality was so skewed, and because
she lied like a cheap rug at the best of times, it was impossible to
gauge what she actually could do and what she couldn't. I filled
out forms saying she couldn't cook for herself, only to have her
aide snort: "Elizabeth, you *know* she can do that just fine. She
just likes to pretend she a queen and be waited on." On the very
rare occasion she agreed to tour a facility, she either looked too
healthy or too sick for their criteria. (Or, once, she screamed
epithets at the director until they asked her to leave.) There's
apparently a tiny slice of time when you are exactly disabled
enough for any given service, and she never seemed to be in
the right place at the right time.

Mostly, she just flat-out refused to consider any plan we put
in front of her. Increasingly desperate, the APS social worker
and I explored every facility in New York that accepted Social
Security or Medicaid subsidies. I had looked into Medicaid eligibility in other states only to have her bark out an ugly, disbe-
lieving laugh—of *course* she wasn't going to leave Manhattan,
how could I be so *stupid*. We found several in Manhattan, and I
arranged for either the social worker or the endlessly amenable
Torsten to accompany her on the required tour before submit-
ting an application. She refused all the tours, sometimes—so
close!—only when her accompanier had arrived in the lobby.

The caseworker showed her brochures, and she scoffed: A shared refrigerator? *Hardly*. Brooklyn? *Not on your life*. The roller coaster of hope and defeat was wearing on us all.

I reminded myself sternly that for someone with agoraphobia, the idea of leaving a home of thirty-five years had to be a level of terrifying I couldn't comprehend. But it seemed that more was at play; every time I approached her about a new assisted living facility, she retorted that she had a month's rent in cash ready for the landlord, everything was fine, and I should butt out. None of us could figure out if she didn't understand or wouldn't admit that she was now three full years in the hole.

I knew we were headed for chaos when she fired Julia, her beloved aide. She'd fired a number of them over the years. This was one way in which she wasn't unusual; elderly people often resent what they see as an intrusion on their privacy and try to refuse the help they don't want to admit they need. Home health-care aides move around a lot. But Julia had been there for four years. In her way, she had loved my mother. (Or, at the least, had allowed herself to be yelled at a lot, which in my mother's orbit is more or less the same thing.) She had fetched her hundreds of rotisserie chickens, shared a thousand Hershey's bars, mopped up daily cigarette ashes, and ferried her down to housing court, oxygen tank and all. But one day, with no warning, my mother started raging at her about napping in the living room. She called the agency and told them never to allow Julia back, and then she called the police. Julia called me from the street, stunned, after being escorted from the building by the cops.

"What is she *doing*, Elizabeth?" she asked plaintively. "I've been working for that woman for four years! I've done everything for her! And now there's police taking me out of the building, and my supervisor at the agency just called and told me I'm fired! What am I gonna do?"

My codependent side opened my mouth to offer to send a check, and then my fury-at-the-lawsuit side, bigger and scalier, reared up through my throat and throttled it back down. "I just don't know, Julia," I said honestly. "If you want to give me your supervisor's contact information, I'll write her a letter saying my mother is emotionally volatile and has fired a lot of aides in her time. I'm sorry this happened to you. I'm so sorry. She's just . . . she's vicious."

"You do that, Elizabeth!" she yelled—Julia's natural speaking voice was a decibel or two above your average helicopter taking off, useful for working with the elderly. "OK. OK, I'm going home to my babies. You be well. Be well."

The court evaluator called me back. The case was over. The judge, perched on the couch in my mother's living room during a "bedside hearing," had offered my mother what the evaluator wonderingly called a sweetheart deal—he would wipe away all of her debt, now nearly in the six figures, if she would agree to a plan toward starting to pay it again. She'd laughed at him and insisted there was no problem, she had a full month's rent saved; all these people should get out of her apartment and leave her *alone*. His kindness spurned, the judge threw up his hands.

"Mrs. Scheier is tangential, confused, and does not seem to understand the severity of her situation," said the evaluator's report. "She has no plan for how to care for herself and will not accept any housing offer that has been made to her." They were out of ideas, too.

There was some comfort in the knowledge that even professionals who dealt with these issues every day were stymied by my mother. Again, I soothed myself: *This isn't just you. You're not crazy. You're not making this up.* I consulted friends. I narrated the events to Arie, straining to present them neutrally. "This isn't normal, right?" I pressed. "I'm not just making up this concern about the kids? I'm not somehow failing her?" His eyebrows raised to his senatorial hairline, he reassured me: I was not.

But I was failing her, of course. I had been the only person left who was willing to put up with her. And here I was, cutting her loose. I shuttled between self-excoriation and a shameful glee at the thought of finally being free of caring for her.

A few weeks later, a terse voice mail from the guardian: the eviction had gone through. The marshals had arrived, drilling through the lock when she wouldn't answer the door, and the movers were throwing her things into boxes. The caseworker had packed her immediate possessions into a single suitcase, tucked an envelope of family photos into her own purse for safekeeping, and bundled her into a waiting car, leaving the silent apartment behind them. My mother was going to the Franklin Women's Intake Shelter in the Bronx.

CHAPTER 14

Gimme Shelter

The irony of my mother living in a homeless shelter didn't escape me.

For seventeen years I'd hoisted myself into the driver's seat of a rickety, rubber-and-chicken-soup-smelling Coalition for the Homeless van every Wednesday night and followed a predetermined route from Saint Bart's in Midtown East, where volunteers loaded giant gray insulated tubs, crates of milk and oranges, and clear trash bags of bagels into the back. We barreled down the FDR to the parking lot outside the housing court, where elderly women speaking Cantonese and wielding lychee-flavored hard candies swarmed the van; they spurned the soup but wanted the milk and oranges for their grandchildren, and the bagels, plain only. Then down Broadway all the way to South Ferry, where in the deepest winter and hottest summer a sentry would run into the ferry terminal to tell bike messengers and odd jobbers that *the van* was there. Around the tip of the island to Madison Square Garden, where fights were most likely to break out and where soup was often thrown; and finally, the jog to Penn Station, where drowsy men and women rousted themselves from their perches in the waiting rooms to come upstairs. And I looked at them and thought: How did you get here? What went wrong? You were falling, and the safety net had holes so big you fell right through. You had problems you couldn't solve on your own, and your family or your friends didn't have the resources, or the wherewithal, or enough patience to handle them. And now here you are.

And now I was the one whose patience was gone. I was the abandoner. In a former armory in the Bronx, my diminished, greasy-haired, hollow-cheeked mother was shuffling from cafeteria to sidewalk to the bedroom she shared with six other women. I have been inside shelters and SROs to drop off food, and trust me, you wouldn't send a dog you liked to one. But there she was.

She somehow stuck it out there for five full weeks. She called a few days in, on my birthday, and rushed off the phone insisting that everything was fine, *fine*; the social worker was arranging her placement, and she'd be all set up soon. I got off the phone and looked at Arie disbelievingly, hope rising in my chest like a cloud of cinnamon; could this finally be the solution? Were we in the clear?

Ha. Ha*ha*. The caseworker called an hour later. Could I get my mother to listen to reason? She'd been offered appointments at assisted living facilities, but dismissed each for an increasingly bizarre list of reasons. I had thought that once the eviction went through, she would accept the reality of the situation. I was convinced that once the safety line to the apartment she so rarely left was severed, she would panic and agree to the options she'd so scornfully refused, acting as if we were all crazy for even suggesting them—Brooklyn! High cabinets! A communal fridge!—knowing that the reality of a shelter was so much worse. Neither her story nor the social worker's story seemed entirely plausible. Obviously everything wasn't fine, as she claimed, and obviously no one would really turn down safe, free housing because she had to share a fridge like the social worker said, would she? *Would* she? I had no idea who or what to believe.

I felt an atavistic urge to get in the car and just go pick her up, get her out of there. Arie and I had gone around the same conversation a thousand times over the last year: What then? She wouldn't consent to any form of housing we could afford, she couldn't stay near our children long-term, and she would see no doctor other than Jackass, who had sworn to a judge that his patient—gasping away on her oxygen tank, barely able to walk, unable or unwilling to admit the severity of her situation—was in "perfect health" and should be left in her apartment under his care. We could empty our retirement accounts and the kids' college funds to rent her a new apartment or pay off the landlord and keep her in hers—for a while, anyway—but with the eyes of the court on her, it might do more harm than good. Formalized support would likely have invalidated her Medicaid eligibility, which paid for the aides who made sure she didn't fall in the bathtub and checked that she was taking her medications. Replacing that care ourselves, the thousands every month plus her rent, would bankrupt us quickly and she would be right back where she started. "How do people *do* this who aren't insanely wealthy?" I raged to Arie, who shook his head over the spreadsheets we built and rebuilt, trying to find a way.

"There's no good answer here," he finally said. "There's no good ending to this story. She's elderly, she's sick, and she's just sane enough that legally she gets to make her own decisions, even if they land her in a homeless shelter. I think . . ." He tapped a few keys, frowned. "I think the best that we can do at this stage is find the least worst option."

The least worst option was Medicaid or Social Security–subsidized assisted living. And she wouldn't fucking *go*. Every time, we came back around to the same conclusion: allowing the crisis to unfold was the only way to get her to agree to a safer, sustainable situation. And I sat on my hands.

She called most days, increasingly manic, not asking for help, but issuing demands. I was to write a check for an oddly specific and large amount of money made out to the Jackass Doctor, which she would retrieve. When I told her it would be a cold day in hell before I had any dealings with him, she amended her order: I could make it out to her and send it to his office, and she would sign it over to him. She did not seem to understand that this suggestion was not an improvement.

She changed strategy. She started calling more often, her voice barely perceptible through the pay phone—I suspected she'd lost her dentures or didn't have a good place to clean them, and her shapeless mouth couldn't form clear syllables—with the hours that it was acceptable for me or Arie to drive down and pick her up and bring her to a hotel. Manhattan only, she was quick to specify. The Upper West Side, preferably. (Never mind that neither I nor my husband have ever been able to afford to live in Manhattan as adults.) Stalling, I asked where she planned or wanted to go long-term; *that's not to be discussed*, she told me haughtily. But I should come, and I should bring a credit card and my checkbook. She hung up before I could answer, whether because she was running out of change or because she didn't want to believe I would say no, I couldn't say.

One Monday morning, I got a call from an unfamiliar number; sure it would be another borrowed cell phone, I took a deep breath, steeled myself, and answered. To my shock, it was one of the shelter social workers, calling me from home on her day off.

"Is there anything you can do to convince your mother to comply with our rules?" she asked.

I tried not to laugh. Clearly she hadn't known her very long. "Rules like what?"

"Well, she won't shower, and it's been a few weeks; the smell of urine is getting strong."

This shook me. My mother had always been fastidious about cleanliness. "She might be afraid of falling," I said doubtfully.

"We have shower chairs, Ms. Scheier," said the social worker. "I used to be a home health-care aide. I told her I'd help. I got changed and put on the rubber gloves, we were all ready to go, and then she changed her mind. Just started shaking her head and went back to her room."

"Mom, why aren't you showering? Do you not feel safe?" I asked, the next time she called. The wheezing over the phone got worse, stringy and wet. "I'm *showering*, Elizabeth! Of course I am! Now *listen* to me. I need *money*. Have you rented me an apartment yet?"

Of course I believed the social worker over her, but I couldn't wrap my mind around that story either. Was this a question of vulnerability—Did it feel too dangerous to get undressed? Was she just so far gone that basic hygiene seemed unnecessary? Did she really believe that she actually *had* taken that shower?

Convinced that the guardian was stealing from her, she refused to talk about any more assisted living placements. She would not countenance living anywhere but Manhattan, so an apartment anywhere we could afford—as dubious as I was that she could live independently—was out. I called my aunt and uncle for the first time in my adult life, hoping they might agree to visit her in a placement near their Arizona home, and that she might see that as an acceptable compromise. They declined in no uncertain terms. "We love her, honey," my aunt said. "But we're not in such good health, and your mother—she's a lot." I couldn't argue with that. And I'd already ruled out my own home. Only a monster would let her mother stay at a homeless shelter.

I was now that monster.

✦ ✦ ✦

During one of her screaming fits in my early twenties, she threatened suicide, a threat so common from her it barely raised an eyebrow. "You can't," I said offhandedly, trying to bring the hysterical tone of the conversation down. "I can't have *two* parents who killed themselves." Silence; and then she never threatened it again. The fact that her suicide might affect other people—the real suicide, not just the manipulation of the threat—seemed not to have occurred to her, and for whatever reason, that idea sank like a stone in quicksand.

In the shelter, it seemed, she was committing suicide by omission. Her only hospital visit in decades had been when a serious UTI clouded her mind and challenged her breathing. My friend Claire's father had died from long-term complications of a UTI;

it's not an unusual way to go for older people, with their mobility and hygiene challenges. And yet she'd stopped bathing. She had been largely incontinent for years; wasn't her own smell bothering her? Was this a protest? Was it a demand? Was she just beyond understanding what was happening?

My memories of my mother's body are fraught. I remember the softness of her arms holding me, and the smell of her skin—Emeraude and Marlboro Reds. I thought I was mistaken about my memory of breastfeeding—surely I had been too young—until my godmother Shannon told me, eyebrows nearly to her hairline, that my mother nursed me until I was four years old. I remember the smell of her warm hair permeating the apartment as she blew it dry to the tinny intro of the 1010 WINS traffic report; the crepey fabric of her cheeks when she got old; the firm crack of her hand across my head when I misbehaved. The way her body ballooned to two hundred pounds when she began living on Mallomars and Hershey's bars; the slackness of her skin when she lost it all because her dentures hurt too much to eat; the heft of her at her heaviest when I'd wrestled her off the floor onto which she'd fallen the day before, slick with shit.

Her body betrayed her as much as her mind, and fueled by rage she couldn't control, it betrayed me too. And now that body was living in a shelter, filthy, stinking, and in need of somewhere to land.

Detritus

Nothing makes you want to clear your own clutter like the sight of all someone's possessions, from wedding album to wheelchair to half-empty box of baking soda, thrown haphazardly into a single metal cage. I took the six a.m. bus up to New York, vibrating with nervous energy and sweating from every pore in the ninety-five-degree heat. Two men from the storage facility caught sight of Alexa and Yumi coming in to meet me, and came up on a cargo elevator the size of a classroom to help wiggle the boxes out from the furniture, piled three deep. It was immediately obvious that there was no way the junkers were going to fit the furniture on a single truck, and that the boxes—the giant kind meant for pillows and plastic toys, as tall as my rib cage—were too many and too tall to fit on the U-Haul I'd rented. The storage facility functioned more like an eviction impound lot, and I had to get everything out of there in one go. There was no time for sentimentality.

I unzipped my bag and handed around scissors and rolls of packing tape, and we each sliced open a box top and started consolidating.

I'd known eviction crews wouldn't exactly be white-gloving it—we were lucky that New York is famously tenant-friendly, and an evicting landlord can't just toss your stuff on the street— but I hadn't thought about just how shitty a packing job can be when the movers aren't working for the movee. Drawers had been upended and dumped in wholesale. Nothing had been wrapped, so everything that could break, broke. Clothes were tangled in, hangers and all. You could see how they'd moved through the apartment, room by room; this box contained the contents of her desk, that one the silverware drawer, the other a pile of glass shards of unknown provenance. One box held half-empty condiment bottles that had been sitting in an un-air-conditioned storage space in July. One held her laundry bag with the dirty laundry still in it. One held dozens of her pill bottles, years and years of expired Ativan and Wellbutrin, half-full.

The pathos was wincingly heavy-handed. The box containing the contents of her dresser also held her jewelry box, a fussy affair with a dozen little drawers that I'd picked out at a flea market as a child. Her jewelry was gone—taken with her or given away, I hoped—but an open bag of M&M's had been thrown in on top and then jostled around, so every drawer I opened revealed a jaunty pile of candy. Life as freshman creative writing assignment.

Yumi whooped victoriously. "Papers! I think this must be the file cabinet." I peered into the box. A swamp of coupons, prescription inserts, what looked like a pile of old letters. "Victory!" I fist-pumped. The truth was somewhere in those boxes, and I was determined to unearth it—literally and met-

aphorically. "Liz, what the . . . ?" Alexa held up a Ziploc bag
full of opera gloves, shaped for child-sized hands, and a pile
of beat-up 20s-era cloches, trailing chic veils. "Ruth's," I said
grimly. "Just throw them in the box. I'll figure it out later."

Hours later—hours after I'd promised my kind, dusty
friends that we'd be done—the truck was full, the boxes packed
to the brim and muscled up into the U-Haul. Alexa and Yumi
waved me off, looking forlornly after the truck. I prayed that
if I was going to hit something, it would be after they were
safely out of sight. The driver's-side mirror was broken, and
unhelpfully displayed either the side of the van or two lanes to
the left. There were no shocks, and with every Bronx pothole
I jounced up half a foot.

The skies opened when I hit Maryland. A few drops at
the tollbooth, steady rain and a darkening sky on the other
side, and halfway onto the bridge lightning seared the horizon and the wind came up fast, blowing the truck—its broad
side acting like the sail of a ship—across two lanes of blessedly
slow traffic. My hands crabbed onto the wheel, I babbled one
long, constant prayer and counted down the minutes. When
I finally pulled into a miraculous empty space in front of the
house, Arie shot out the front door and helped me uncrunch
myself from behind the wheel. "I should have gone with you,"
he said, clearly angry at himself.

"And done what with the kids, strapped them to the roof
of the truck?" He shook his head, speechless, and rattled the
lock on the enormous truck, testing the shank. "This is such
a mess," I said, my voice wavering, and he put his arm around
my shoulders and we went inside.

We spent the next two days unpacking and repacking the
contents of my mother's life, eager to get in the Goodwill run

before we had to return the truck. I had nightmare visions of my house overtaken by dusty, broken-glass-filled boxes forever, her life overtaking ours, her trash becoming our own. Twenty-seven boxes of donations went right back on the truck. We kept a few useful kitchen items, a colander, an ice cream scoop. Bags and bags and bags of trash, much of it broken or filthy or both, went right out the back door. As I sorted through towering piles of her mother's 1940s and her own 1980s paperback best sellers, a full set of the Yale Shakespeare, and histories broad and narrow, I thought ruefully back to my publishing days, the book lovers' rhapsodies about the smell of old books. Ha. Unless you're keeping your treasured books in the temperature-controlled bliss of the Smithsonian, they're trash waiting to happen. Half of them flaked to papery shards in my hands.

So much was missing that didn't make sense. Most of her battered stainless steel flatware was gone, leaving only two salad forks and an impressive pile of wooden takeout chopsticks. I found the shards of just a few dishes, and one salad plate miraculously whole; the rest were gone. No sign of the tiny metal tins that had lived in her breakfront for years, containing the ashes of my childhood dog and her ancient cat. Maybe she'd tossed it all. Over the last year she had taken to shedding years' worth of hoarding, as careless as she had once been grasping. Packages began to arrive at my door, some with notes, some without. A sheaf of random photographs. My long-dead grandmother's will. Once, notably, an unmarked packet of my own baby teeth, which clicked into my palm like bones. I jumped and shrieked like an actress in a grade-B horror movie.

My childhood things fared better, having been packed long ago. A Bankers Box of my dollhouse furniture, painstakingly collected over years, individually wrapped in paper towels. A pile of my childhood dresses, lovingly ironed and folded. (*Ironed*, for the love of all that's holy; for a *two*-year-old.) My Cabbage Patch dolls, naked and folded floppily, toes to bulbous face. Four miniature Maurice Sendak books, immediately claimed by my toddlers, who clutched their little red books with Mao-ish fervor.

A hardback series of Mark Twain: back in the box. Four-count-'em-four tea strainers, from a coffee household: back in the box. A faux fur coat I'd never seen: back in the box. Piles of half-full, souring condiment bottles: into the trash. Piles of broken vases: trash. Socks and underwear and single gloves: trash trash trash. I was overwhelmed by the sheer weight of possessions. I thought back to myself as a bookish child, obsessed with the Little House on the Prairie books, wondering how people traveled from place to place like turtles, all their possessions more or less on their backs, and as I looked around at the boxes full of items unlooked at for years, I felt a little sick.

And yet I feared missing something. In the movie version of my life, would the audience watch, groaning, as I tossed an unassuming paperback with an overlooked photo of my father used as a bookmark? Would a pile of papers include a squirreled-away marriage certificate? Was one of these books really a journal? I shook out every book and checked every pocket.

My husband isn't a pack rat, but stuff doesn't bother him. Left to his own devices, I think every item that came in the front door would find a place, somewhere, and live there forever. We live in a house, the first one I've ever lived in, and the existence of our attic is a constant marvel to me: a dedicated space, airless and unfit for human habitation, but a place where we can just *leave* stuff. I'm happy leaving a carefully curated box of memories or two, and there are some seasonal items where I see the advantage—the kids' holiday books and toys, our swim gear, the suitcases—but every time I climb those stairs I see the houses I saw flattened and spilling piles of undifferentiated trash after Hurricane Sandy, Caitlin's childhood home burned to ash by a wildfire as she sat in middle school homeroom, a phone video of Lauren holding up her childhood journals to the camera in her Katrina-leveled home, the pages stuck together with mold, her expression unreadable behind the gas mask. Now to those images I could add all of this *stuff*, both the treasured and the dropped-there, piled carelessly into boxes and carted off to the dump. I ached to go through it with a gimlet eye and a firm hand, and get all the most necessary items out before they were taken from us.

Somewhere in here was the document box Yumi had found: the holy grail, the contents of the avocado-green filing cabinet that had sat at the back of her closet for decades. It was always locked. I knew this because on the rare occasions my mother left the house, I searched everywhere I could—desk, nightstand, closets—for some kind of clue as to where the fuck we had come from, how the fuck we had gotten where we were, and what the fuck—what the *fuck*—had become of my glaringly absent father. I was sure that somewhere in there was a birth certificate, a wedding photo, a favorite sweatshirt, some damn thing that would show immutably who he was, or at the very least, that he had ever been there. By high school I had begun to feel like Athena sprung whole from Zeus's forehead, no second parent required.

I rolled my shoulders, took a deep breath, and started opening files.

She wrote a dozen wills between the early 70s and the early

2000s. From them I found out the name of her first mother-in-law, the owner of the hope chest that now sits in my dining room. I found out that she took her abusive second husband's name, leaving yet another name behind. "Judith Miller" was not anyone I knew or had heard of, and yet that was her legal name for most of my life. One will expressly stated that Merrill should get nothing, citing his abuse; another named Torsten as a second recipient of all her estate, should I predecease both of them.

I thought of calling him and cheerfully informing him that should he decide to kill me, he could stand to inherit *tens of dollars*! Or, looked at another way—$70,000 in debt to her landlord! A steal! I restrained myself.

Other discoveries included:

- The delayed birth certificate she had apparently acquired for me the year I entered college. If you don't file for a birth certificate within the first year of a child's life, you have to petition the court to get it done. The parent has to show up in person, which I'd thought would be a bridge too far. Thinking she'd never followed through, I had spent dozens of hours during my layoff trying to assemble the needed identification, stymied at every turn—elementary school records lost in Hurricane Sandy, documents my mother thought vaguely might be "somewhere"—and had finally given up in frustration. She'd had the damn thing for more than a decade, and had either forgotten or had been keeping it hostage.
- A naming certificate for me, signed by a rabbi famous for his thoughtful writing on abortion, at a synagogue in Bay Ridge—at least an hour away from my mother by cab, a Brooklyn neighborhood in which I would have previously

staked my life that she had never set foot. There are dozens of synagogues in Manhattan; several were in walking distance of her apartment. Why there? "Maybe she . . . consulted with that rabbi," suggested Arie delicately. "Glad he wasn't too convincing," I grumbled.

• One of those "stories for my grandchildren" books, written by—mysteriously—my mother's biological uncle, a man she got in touch with only after the death of her birth father. It is chatty, funny, and occasionally raunchy—a little strange, given that he wrote it to a twelve-year-old girl whom he had only met as a small child. I do feel for my mother, befriending her uncle later in life to tell her about the father she never knew. I don't know how she could have lived through a similarly timed absence—although it was an abandonment, not a loss—and come out of it thinking that the best way to manage my father's death was to obscure every known fact about him and make some fake ones up to take their place. But she did.

• An exchange of letters with our downstairs neighbor, a lovely woman with airy blond hair and a soft voice. Susan acknowledges receipt of my mother's voice mail but notes acerbically that, given my mother's screaming public tirade at her daughter after the daughter innocently called her by her first name, she is not necessarily excited to speak with her in person about it. My mother's eight-page draft response (Kept for . . . ? Pride? Regret? Who knows?) goes on to excoriate both the young woman and the mother who raised her, and inexplicably contains three intermediate pages bragging about my high school volunteer projects. (She also claims, hilariously, that my husband called her "Mrs. Scheier" until the day we married, after which he

called her "Mom." This is total fiction. Luckily for my husband, he hasn't had occasion to call her much of anything.)
Susan's response points out that it's all very nice, but that
she doubts I'd be too thrilled about this comparison; I burst
into humiliated tears, and only barely stopped myself from
looking up her number to call and tell her that I had nothing to do with the whole incident. I am not, I reminded
myself, my mother's keeper.

- And an exchange of letters between her lawyer friend
Don—another person she occasionally suckered into releasing his letterhead into the world on her behalf, like a flock
of flying monkeys—and the upstairs neighbors, an elderly
couple who had had the gall to use a NordicTrack in their
bedroom during daylight hours. The two-page letter
from Don explains their sin in regretful and reserved
tones; I imagine even he did not want to write it, and
that he was badgered or charmed into it. Their response
is quick and severe: "Your letter is basically a recital of
outright lies," they begin, and they go on in that vein. In
the middle of the second page, my heart fell. "We have
lived at 27 W. 96th St. for 28 years in complete har-
mony with our neighbors, the staff, and the owners of the
building. Your client is the only exception, and for her to
scream at us over the intercom in the building's lobby that
'I hope you have a heart attack while exercising' should be
ample proof of her irrationality. It should also be noted
that during all of the years that she has lived below us,
we have never complained of the distress caused us by
Ms. Scheier's constant screaming at her daughter, widely
heard and remarked on by other tenants. At one point,
this verbal barrage was of such intensity that it brought

the aforementioned Mr. Silver up to her apartment in the middle of the night to make sure no physical harm was being done."

Well.

My head buzzed, and an angry red mottle rushed up my neck and to my hairline. I pressed my cool hands to my forehead and sobbed once, more in humiliation and fury than in sadness. I remembered that night. My mother's voice when she answered the door, tense with interruption, and Mr. Silver's cool tone: "We heard a loud bang and wanted to make sure that the refrigerator hadn't fallen over."

The noise he'd heard was me slamming my bedroom door, hard. At the time, I thought his visit was a passive-aggressive complaint—*keep it down up here, kid.* And maybe it was. Or maybe, as the self-righteous NordicTrack enthusiast had reported, a halfhearted attempt at tracking what was going on a few feet over his head. I remembered Gretchen's epiphany over beers—*Mom came with me on all the playdates so I would never be alone with Mrs. Scheier*—and was swamped with an inexplicable, searing embarrassment. They had all been watching, and judging. The neighbors had sat in their identical floor-plan apartments up and down the line, TVs turned down and conversation stopped in midsentence, listening to her scream. Their family dinners had been interrupted. Their silent, companionate reading. Their own (quieter) arguments.

And but for that one abbreviated visit, they did nothing.

The letter writers say nothing about hearing her hit me. I have to hope that if they had, they would have overcome their own distress to come downstairs. There's no law against yelling at your kid. But I need to believe that if they had known what was really going on, they would have intervened, as the police who flinched back when she brained me against a doorframe did not.

This rocked my narrative. Life with Judith Scheier made sense, barely, if you understood it as a life lived in isolation, a locked panic room in the middle of a boisterous, crowded city. We were largely alone (Exhibit A: mystery father) and nearly off the grid (Exhibit B: no birth certificate; Exhibit C: fake Social Security number). With no one there to witness, our lives could continue unspooling with no voices of sanity to intervene.

But there had been eyes on us. There had been ears. And those silent observers changed the whole story. That apartment wasn't a panic room. It was a fishbowl.

In the endless pile of cracked and shattering books was a newer hardcover, dust jacket removed. I flipped to the title page, threw my head back, and howled. For years, I had been thinking desultorily of hunting down a copy of Christine Ann Lawson's *Understanding the Borderline Mother*, a social worker's help guide for adult children. It was long out of print, and there was always something better to spend $80 on than a used copy of a book I didn't even know if I'd like. I had read *Stop Walking on Eggshells*, the bible for people related to people with BPD, and found it smarmy at best and homophobic at worst.

Also, of course, I was a coward. An exhausted one. Reading the book would mean temporarily accepting one of many diagnoses she'd claimed to have, possibly for nothing. It would mean committing to some kind of action to protect myself from her, when just protecting her was tiring enough. I was too engaged in dodging through a burning house to just pick up the damn hose.

But. My mother had bought the book herself, and I was

holding it in my hands. I don't know who she thought the mother of the title was—if she was reading to understand her own relationship with Ruth, or if she was trying to see herself through my eyes. (She owned a number of well-thumbed books with titles like *Toxic Parents*, a humbling discovery that always made my eyes sting.) Whatever she hoped to get out of it, she gave up early. The bookmark was tucked into page thirteen.

I read the whole thing in a few nights, highlighting so much I turned whole pages yellow. Arie, who had never seen me so much as dog-ear a page, eyed me with wonder from the next pillow over. Lawson characterizes the types of borderline mothers as waifs who need rescuing, hermits who need soothing, queens who need subjects, and witches who need something to burn. I rolled my eyes at the fairy-tale language, but her descriptors were spot-on, and I saw both the queen and the witch in my mother. "Children who grow up with borderline mothers live in a make-believe world that is neither fiction nor fantasy," Lawson wrote, and I fist-pumped jubilantly.

"Read it to me," Arie said, and I did.

"You see," I said, half-laughing and half-crying. "This isn't just me. I didn't make this up."

He shook his head disbelievingly. "Of course you didn't. I know that."

He knew, but I hadn't been sure. It was world exploding to see my experience described on the page, and to see it understood as not normal. My mother wasn't just strict, or tough on me, or a yeller. She was inherently nonfunctional in the world. She was so fucking sick. And she had set us both on fire.

CHAPTER 16

Mermaid Manor

She stretched those two allowable weeks in the intake shelter into five. And then she disappeared.

The guardian left me a voice mail telling me my mother had finally—*finally*—had an interview at an assisted living facility. I called her back the next day to ask how it had gone.

"Oh, your mother's been transferred!" she said brightly.

". . . To the ALF?" I asked. Silence. The transfer paperwork didn't say, and she didn't know. Somehow, a seventy-nine-year-old woman who used a walker and a portable oxygen tank, and who had a guardian and the shelter social worker looking out for her, had just walked off.

The shelter's main number rang endlessly. Dead end. OK. I called the guardian back.

"I'll call them and see if they have her," I said. "Can you give me the name and number of the facility?"

"Well, I don't have the phone number, but it's called Mermaid Manor."

I'm not ashamed to report that I giggled, a little hysterically. "*Mermaid Manor? Really?*"

The guardian laughed. "It's in Coney Island, on Mermaid Avenue. I bet your mom gets a kick out of that!" *I bet she's already decked a nurse*, I thought.

I called Mermaid Manor and kept hitting zero until I got through to a person. On a hunch, I didn't explain the situation—I wouldn't even have known where to start—just asked politely to speak to Judith Scheier.

"*Who?*" yelled a voice over the din.

"Judith Scheier?" I tried again, heart sinking.

"Judith—oh, *Judy*! The new one. Hang on." The phone clunked down and my jaw dropped. No one had called my mother Judy since the first grade, and sure as shit almost no one had called her by her first name in my hearing without getting royally reamed out. What brave new world was this?

The phone clunked up. "*Hello?*" my mother's voice yelled. My stomach bottomed out with relief. I hadn't realized how unnerving it had been to talk to her only through staticky pay phones.

"Hi, Mom. How are you doing?"

"Oh, it's *you*!" She was delighted. "How *are* you?"

"I'm fine, Mom. How are you? How's Mermaid Manor?"

"Oh, it's *very* nice. The people are lovely. And I only have one roommate!"

God help that roommate, I thought. She sounded better already; she had her dentures back, or had been reminded to wear them, and the chatter of voices in the background sounded so much homier than the echoing halls of the shelter.

"Did they come pick you up?"

"Yes, they sent a van, and Elizabeth, the driver was *so nice*. He has a son just your age who . . ." and off she went on the story of Earl the van driver, while I gave Arie a thumbs-up as he tried to keep the kids from chewing on the rug.

"So you're going to stay awhile?" I finally broke in.

She huffed. "Oh, *Elizabeth*. Don't you worry about me. This is none of your concern. I can take care of myself—"

"OK! OK. Just asking. Well, happy settling in, Mom, call me if you need anything, OK?"

"Bring the babies to see me!" she trilled.

I ended the call. Arie was standing next to me, eyebrows raised. "Well," I said gruffly. "We were trying to find afford-able senior housing. So I guess: least worst option?"

"Least worst option," he assured me, and I burst into tears of relief on his shoulder.

She called me every couple of days, or I called her. Most days, she complained about the roommate, the food, the fact that she wasn't allowed to smoke in her room. (She did anyway, and bribed her roommate with Hershey's bars to go out and buy more cigarettes for her.) But there was a different tone to her complaining. She wasn't hysterical, and didn't sound on the verge of running out into the street and angling for the near-est oncoming truck. Maybe, I figured, she'd gotten her med-ication back. Or maybe the presence of nurses and the lesser din of a nursing home was giving her hair-trigger brain some peace. I started to think that maybe the change could be per-manent; maybe she could get used to living somewhere else. Maybe, after all these years, she was finally living somewhere where medical staff were nearby should she fall again, or as she inevitably, inexorably declined. Somewhere we could afford, with the sizable Social Security subsidy. And from which she couldn't be evicted.

She lasted at Mermaid Manor for exactly two weeks.

The Jackass Doctor came to visit her, and on my warning, they turned him away. The next morning, she scooted up to the social worker, her butt balanced precariously on the bar of her walker; she couldn't walk, she claimed. She was in too much pain, and her feet wouldn't work. She wheezed and peered over her bifocals; the social worker, no fool, quickly called an ambulance. She had liked my mother at the beginning, but was stunned by the quick turnaround in her attitude: "I thought she was this nice tiny old lady from Belle Harbor!" she lamented to me. "Now she says . . . I can't even repeat what she says!" *You and me both, lady*, I thought grimly. *You and me both.*

Once in the ambulance, she convinced them to take her north from the spur of Coney Island all the way up through Brooklyn, across the bridge, and up half the narrow column of Manhattan to the Upper West Side, and checked herself into Mount Sinai West. There are a dozen hospitals between the one and the other, any one of which the EMTs could have taken her to. Maybe she genuinely was having trouble walking. Maybe this was her way of getting back to her beloved Manhattan, from which she had been removed at drill point. She was not going to be thwarted by stupid *laws*, or stupid *rules*, or stupid *lack of any assets or income at all*. She was going back to the noise and the bustle, even if she had to look down on it from a hospital window. Maybe. But I thought I knew what she was looking for: she wanted the Jackass Doctor. If Muhammad couldn't go to the mountain, the mountain was going to rise up and go to Muhammad.

CHAPTER 17

Checking In

Doctors started calling in the morning and just kept on calling. I tracked her progress through the system by the title of the person on the phone. She started out in the emergency room (an ER doctor) and was checked into the rheumatology ward (resident); she refused to allow anyone near her (social worker) and screamed assault when they tried (psychiatrist). She told them I was coming to pick her up and rent her an apartment (social worker again). I called patient services (account manager) and told them to kick the Jackass Doctor onto the street if he tried to show up. A former aide named Roslyn, who'd left the agency for a job at a nursing home, came by after work to turn my mother with gentle hands and give her a sponge bath.

A second social worker—Really, I was going to rent her an apartment on the Upper West Side? I explained as gently as I could that I was not. Another resident—Her oxygen was low, she was still smoking, how could she be smoking in a hospital? Could I talk her out of it? I choke-laughed. A psychiatrist— Was she a suicide risk? WHAT DO YOU THINK, I didn't yell. She was living in Mount Sinai like it was a Motel 6. Who goes to a hospital and refuses to see a doctor? Judith Scheier, ladies and gentlemen.

A new resident called me, confused; she was confronted with a hostile elderly woman who had demanded to come to the ER and then refused to allow anyone to touch her. "She said it would be . . . assault?" she said tentatively. *Listen*, I wanted to say, *settle in. It's only going to get weirder from here*. Without examining her, they had no way of figuring out what to do. They agreed to send her back and made the call to transport. I breathed a sigh of relief and emailed the Mermaid Manor social worker to let her know Mom was on her way back.

I lay in bed that night, Arie breathing softly next to me, and felt the cold shaky rush of long-held adrenaline leaving my body. It was going to be OK. The long nightmare was almost over. Even she couldn't thwart the system's gears forever; finally, she had landed in care that was competent if not cushy, and where she would be safe.

And yet the next morning, an email from the bowels of Mermaid Manor: "Your Mom is not back yet. Could you please let me know what's going on." Of course. Of *course* it wasn't that simple. At my desk two hundred miles away, I banged my forehead softly against my monitor.

I called Irina the social worker back. She had no idea where Mom was. *How do you lose an old woman who can't walk by herself*, I didn't yell. Bless her, by that afternoon she had tracked down the hospital's social worker and gotten Mom's room number. I was tired of bewildered silence on the other end of the phone.

I wanted to know what the ever-living fuck was going on. I was already on my way home, and I ducked into an alcove in the Metro entrance and dialed. In retrospect I should have waited until I got home to somewhat more comfortable surroundings, but when your missing crazy mother washes up somewhere with a number that accepts incoming calls, you dial that phone fast.

I gave the switchboard operator her name; they put me through to her room, where she sounded full of beans and just delighted with everything. "ELIZABETH!" she trumpeted. "How delightful to hear from you! How are my grandchildren?"

Not homeless, I thought grimly, *so that's something*. "They're fine, Mom. How are you? What brought you to the hospital?"

"WELL." I heard a shuffling; the crackle and squawk of the TV turned off abruptly. "Here's what I need you to do, honey: I need you to come to New York today or tomorrow. And I need you to rent me a one-bedroom apartment, Manhattan, obviously. Nothing huge; a bedroom, a small kitchen, and a living room. Oh, and it has to be within a block of Central Park, of course."

Sparks crackled in my head. She never left her bedroom. It didn't matter if that room was in a Fifth Avenue palace or a concrete bunker at the center of the earth. I slotted in my headphones and quickly googled as she went on—"average rent one bedroom upper west"—and groaned. She was still going: ". . . You need to buy some furniture—a bed, a small couch, a dining table, all that kind of thing—and you'll also need to bring some cash. Roslyn will have to go buy flatware, glasses, all that stuff. I need to replace everything!"

"Mom. Mom. Mommmmmm." I brought her spiel to a

halt. "I just looked it up. Apartments like the one you want rent for an average of $4,100 a month."

A pause.

"For WHAT?"

"They rent for more than four thousand dollars."

She would not be deterred. "Well, we'll just have to find something that costs about a quarter of that! And you'll only have to pay for the first few months, anyway; then Medicaid will pay for it." I had kept from laughing so far, but this was too much for me; I let out a strangled half-chortle, half-moan. I heard her draw herself up, offended. "Oh, *Elizabeth*. They will. You don't know anything about anything. You don't know anything even about food stamps, but *I* know." *How do you think all your eligibility renewal paperwork got filled out all these years, you disingenuous harridan*, I thought but did not say. I got myself off the phone by promising to look into it, and I got on the Metro, where I rage-cried silently all the way home.

"Well, she needs control over something," Arie said mildly as I related the conversation to him in bed that night, complete with ranting and strangling hand gestures. I knocked my head against his shoulder blade and sighed, comforted by his solidity, and by his laughter at every bizarre statement I repeated. If it was funny, maybe there was a joke in here somewhere; maybe this was less tragedy than bizarro stage play. Maybe it was still possible that the wall would break open and a curtain would slide back and the audience would be revealed, applauding, bells ringing and lights flashing.

A social worker called the next morning. "I'm just the temp!" he said cheerily. "The regular social worker is on vacation. But let's see what we've got here." Papers shuffled. "So your mom came in complaining that she couldn't walk. She definitely won't get out of bed, but that's all we know. What we're really concerned about is her oxygen levels. They're at barely over eighty percent and she won't use a tank. Any idea how to convince her?" I laughed, and he laughed with me, ruefully. He had a Jewish name, and he likely knew how much credence a mother like mine would give to medical instruction.

"Listen, I know you can't tell me much because of HIPAA—" I started.

He chuckled. "Oh, don't worry about *that*! Let's see what the doctor put in the chart." And I sat with mouth open, thumb-typing furiously, as he read her chart aloud to me: Joint and muscle pain. Arthritis. COPD. Bunions. A nebulizer and oxygen tank she wouldn't use. Refused PT. Refused shower. Refused examination.

"So what do you *do* in these cases?" I asked. "She can't just stay there forever, right? What happens now? Do you send her back to Mermaid Manor? Do you call the police?"

"I'll level with you, Ms. Scheier," he said. "We sometimes keep people here for a very, very long time when they have nowhere else to go. You'd be surprised how often that happens. Obviously we want to provide her with medical care, but we're not just going to throw her out on the street. Don't you worry about that."

Wait till she really gets going, I thought sourly. *You'll be the first one waving her out the door.*

When the phone rang again, it was her aide, Roslyn. "Elizabeth!" she shouted into the phone. "Listen, we got to get your mother out of here."

I banged my head softly against the desk. "Yes, well. She

was in the assisted living facility but demanded to go to the hospital. She *had* another place. She wouldn't *stay* there. I'm happy to take any suggestions you have."

"Elizabeth, you *know* I work at the New Jewish Home now." (Point of fact: I did not know that. Come to think of it, I wasn't even sure how Roslyn had my number.) "You just send her *here*. I'll take care of her my*self*. You know I always tell her: I'm her Black daughter. I'll take care of her."

I perked up, ignoring the Black daughter business, a sentiment repeated by enough aides that it was clear it had come from my mother, a tidbit that horrified me. "Oh? Does the New Jewish Home have beds?"

She snorted. "You just let God worry about that, Elizabeth!"

Not wanting to offend, I paused, and then, delicately: "Well. Maybe God and the patient coordinator?"

She laughed. "I'm going to go turn your mother over, Elizabeth. You know she's got bedsores!" And she was gone.

Bedsores, Jesus. I struggled with the image of my mother, old and vulnerable and physically hurting. She had caused so much chaos in my life, even when I was an adult, that I saw her as large and impervious, and I was still afraid of her. It was a rude shock to think of her unable to turn over in her hospital bed. Her charm had kept her afloat this long, but how much longer could that last?

A day passed, then another, then a weekend. The doctors kept calling, and I kept explaining patiently: Yes, she struggled with mental illness. No, I wasn't going to rent her an apartment. Yes, she probably was finding a way to smoke. Yes, even if she couldn't walk. Yes. I know. Yes, she certainly is something.

Roslyn was the second call on Tuesday; she was cheerful, but tired. The third call came in as I was coming home from work, wrestling my virtuous reusable bags of groceries up the steps.

"Can I speak to Elizabeth Scheier, please?"

"Yes, this is she."

"This is Dr. Buddhev from Mount Sinai. I'm calling about your mother. We just need to get a few things squared away. Do you have a minute?"

I hip-checked the door open. "Sure. What can I do for you?"

"Well, we're trying to get some paperwork in order. Your mother has a guardian, is that right?"

I gave her the name of the guardian and of the agency. "They're just financial guardians, though. She doesn't have a full guardian."

"So they can't make medical decisions?"

"Nope. She has a living will, though. Do you need a copy?"

"I—wait a second." The phone clunked down and her voice came through muffled, talking to someone in the room with her. "Yes. I know. I'm on the phone with the daughter now. One minute." The phone crackled up again. "Does she have a DNR?"

I laughed. "Boy, does she. An EMT ignored it once and I thought she was going to pull out his—"

"Ms. Scheier," the doctor said softly. "Your mother's oxygen is very low, and it's falling. It sounds like you can make medical decisions for her. We can intubate her if you tell us to, but we only have a few minutes."

The world whined to a stop and I smelled ozone. A can fell from my hand to the counter. "I'm sorry, I—I think I didn't understand what we were talking about here. I thought we were talking about paperwork."

Her voice was soft. "No."

"So she's—sorry, I'm trying to get a handle on this. Is my mother dying *right now*?"

"We can intubate her, if you think that's what she'd want. But." A beat. "You would have to tell us now."

If I prolonged that woman's life—if I averted the death she'd prayed for daily for decades—she would never forgive me. "No," I said. I choked. "She wouldn't want that."

"I'm going to go into the room now, OK? You'll be on speakerphone."

"OK," I said blindly, my eyes stinging with tears. The phone rustled, and I heard her muffled footsteps. Mechanical beeping, and the fuzz of quiet voices. I heard a coughing sound, a small choke. The doctor spoke softly to the nurses. I hovered over the couch, not sitting. I didn't know what I was supposed to be doing. I turned in fruitless half-circles, put my phone on speaker, took it off. "Can she hear me if I talk?" I got out. There was no answer. Another minute passed, two, four. My cheek grew hot from my oily phone screen, and I put in headphones. A muffled question, and a response.

And silence.

Footsteps, and the crackle of hallway noise. The doctor put the phone back up to her ear. Her soft voice shook slightly, and I thought: *I bet you don't get a lot of deaths in rheumatology.* "Your mother passed very peacefully," she said. "She wasn't fully conscious. She just breathed more and more slowly and shallowly until she was gone. There was no struggle."

"I—OK." I was writing everything down in my journal, taking notes, not knowing what else to do. "What do I have to do now? What do I need to arrange?"

"I can call you back—"

"*No!*" I gulped. "I'm sorry. No. Let's just do this."

I confirmed that she was an organ donor and refused an autopsy. *What're they going to find?* I thought wildly. *A belly full of condom-wrapped heroin? A treasure map? A gunshot wound?* She was an old woman with a wracking cough and a weak heart. Nothing to see here. No more surprises. The doctor gave me her condolences one last time and got off the phone. I hope to hell she kept a bottle in her desk.

When the call disconnected, my podcast turned back on automatically, and Ira Glass's studiedly nebbishy voice squeaked out of the earbuds. I turned it off.

I was still standing in front of the couch, looking out the front window. Late-afternoon summer sun slanted down the street, and the houses and crape myrtles sheened white, overexposed. It felt like time had stopped. Other than a handful of hospital staff, strangers, I was the only one in the world who knew that my mother was dead. Two hundred miles north, strange hands were pulling a sheet up over her face. Someone was recording the time of death on a clipboard. An efficient clutch of nurses was moving from the drama of caring for a sick woman to the logistics of disposing of her body. In everyone else's world, she was still alive. I teetered between wanting to call everyone at once, and wanting to sit for a long time in this tense moment between when I knew and when everyone else did. There is such a short span between death and the arrangements of death. Only a few seconds where there was a nurse and a sheet, and my hand and the phone.

Judith Scheier was dead.

I don't know how it came as a surprise to me. It was a miracle she had made it so long. She'd hardly left her room in decades, and her exercise consisted of shuffling to the bathroom and back. There were years when most of her calories came from six-packs of Hershey's bars and Entenmann's sheet cakes. After smoking up to six packs a day for sixty years, it was a miracle that she had lungs at all, and not just a rib cavity filled up with that horsehair they used to use to insulate attics.

But I *was* surprised. I was shocked. I had thought she would live forever. I had thought we were yoked together for our whole lives, a solid crossbar of need, disappointment, and love keeping us marching, arms' length but never fully apart. I couldn't remember a time when she hadn't been sick, but she had never been dying. She had hit a mortal drop-off from cantankerous to dead in a single day.

I couldn't get Arie on the phone—the train he was on was coming into the station, and he couldn't hear me over the shriek of the wheels—so I texted tersely, "My mother just died." I called Claire, who gasped and cried with me. I looked at my hands, mouth dry, and didn't know what to do with myself. Arie came home sober faced and held me, my face buried in his shoulder. The kids ran around our feet, babbling and yelling, thrilled to be free of the stroller.

"I WANT SELTZER," Rachel yelled. "I WANT STRAW-BERRY I WANT—"

"Kid," said Arie, raising his head. "You gotta learn to read the room."

Later that night, I called her friends, what few there were left in the mostly crossed-out Rolodex I'd rescued from her boxes. There weren't many. A study had crossed my desk that week about the devastating health effect isolation has on elderly people. My mother, the poster child for isolation, shed people like skin cells. They were startling conversations. I was not under any illusions about who my mother was, or about her inability to manage relationships in anything approaching a normal way. But I can't deny how upsetting it was to hear that so many of the people she considered her closest friends were either evidently untouched, or outright confused as to why I was calling them or why I thought they'd want to know. Her isolation was undoubtedly of her own making. But it was hard to hear how completely she'd burned her bridges.

The next morning, when I was sure I'd reached everyone who should get a personal call, I posted on Facebook.

"Judith Scheier, 1939–2019.

"My mother died early last night. To say that I have mixed feelings would be a vast understatement; she was by turns a brilliant, bullheaded, loving, hilarious, rageful, and violent woman. There was no room she didn't light up, and no relationship she didn't blow up to the heavens. She was a chaos monger, but she was MY chaos monger, and I am mourning her loss with the same ferocity with which I once feared her. She had a hard life, and two weeks short of her eightieth birthday, that life is over.

"Man, would she have had something to say about THAT timing.

"We are burying her on Friday morning next to her mother, grateful that she ultimately decided her desire to be buried in a glass coffin on a hilltop 'like Lenin' was more complicated in execution than it would be worthwhile in dramatics. If you are interested in attending the graveside service, please contact Claire Brooks for details.

"*Baruch dayan ha'emet.* May her memory be for a blessing."

Say what you will about social media—and it is, for certain, a place that allows good people to be bad and bad people to be worse—but the outpouring of affection, commiseration, and love was a giant comfort. And a relief. It was no longer just my story. Some long-ago colleagues who'd met her when we fled uptown to her apartment on 9/11 remembered her in the light of that strange, unsettling memory. "I remember first meeting (and being grilled by) your mother more than twenty years ago," said an old boyfriend. From a girl I knew in high school: "'The infamous three [because we counted the dog] . . . are out having a good time. Leave a message and we may call you back.' I'll forever hear her voice on your outgoing answering machine message." (I have no memory of this message, but man, does it ever sound like her.) And a succinct, pithy sound bite from a woman I'd met once at Yom Kippur services and friended on a whim, never to see again: "It is always hard to lose a mother, even if it was also hard to have one."

Mostly, it was odd to know that others remembered her. We had so rarely been in the same room with other people.

A week after she died, I ignored a call from an unknown number. The voice mail was a familiar voice, Sophia, an old friend of hers from La Leche League, of all places, for whom I'd done data entry in my broke twenties. She had called my mother to wish her a happy new year, and had gotten the phone number shutoff message; had Mom moved? I texted her the news, briefly but as kindly as I could, and a moment later the phone rang again. I let it go to voice mail. I am not good on the phone at the best of times, and this was not near the best of times. She was dismayed, and sorry, so sorry. "Elizabeth, your mom . . ." her voice broke. "She saved my life. When we met I was still in this relationship with Nico's father, and she—she saved my life. I miss her. We were out of touch, but I miss her. Love you, honey. Love you."

I thought of the phone cord and the deadbolts, the vanished husband. So many women of that era who put their heads down and shut their mouths. I don't doubt that my mother did coax Sophia out of that relationship in time to save her life, and to save the psyche of her young son. I don't know how she did it—my mother was never much of a cajoler, more of a "don't be a nitwit" hammer in search of a nail—but I believe that she did. This was the Judith Scheier who invited nineteen-year-old staff from the farm where we spent summers to NYC, took them to see *Cats* and taste their first lox at Zabar's. The Judith Scheier who rented rooms to homesick international students who stayed for years, who saw her as their second mother, who wailed in genuine grief when they heard she had died. She was a much better secondary mother than she was a primary one.

I did the math compulsively and came up with shit every time. Assuming that the eviction didn't hasten her death, and that July 30 was the day no matter what else happened, she'd held on to that apartment through thirty years of scrimping for rent and three years of not paying it at all, only to leave it in the last few weeks of her life. If the already snail's-pace court had moved just a little slower, she might have died in her own bed, never spending a day stinking and hungry in a homeless shelter. *Don't think like that*, I told myself. But I couldn't not. I could only rack up the what-ifs. What if I had given her that first month's rent. What if I had threatened the Jackass Doctor away from her. What if I had let her move in with us, keeping both eyes on her hands and their proximity to the kids. What if I had just kept trying.

I will never know for sure why she went to the hospital. Part of me—not the rational part—thinks that she could feel her own death coming and wanted the painkillers. That her fear of a painful death outweighed her hatred of hospitals. I want to believe that even at the end, even unable to walk and surrounded by strangers, she was able to take control of some measure of her life, even if only the place and comfort of its ending. Surely we all deserve that.

CHAPTER 18

I Lift Up My Eyes

Jews bury our dead within three days; the same day, if we can. It's a pragmatic tradition as well as a religious one. We're a desert people, and we don't preserve bodies. So funeral attendees are always a weird hodgepodge of people who you can wait for and the people who could get off work at short notice. One of Arie's best friends was there. A young woman from synagogue who I hadn't spoken to or thought of in years. A single person from my mother's life—a high school friend who cracked us all up with the story of my mother's graduation gift to all her friends: personalized stationery, with every envelope pre-addressed back to her. Alexa and Yumi. Torsten and his wife. Gabriela, who flew in on her pilot husband's miles from North Carolina, green-lipped with the misery of her first trimester. We stood under the cemetery's entry arch waiting for the rabbi, telling jokes, introducing people to each other. I couldn't remember the synagogue woman's name, and panicked. *You are not a host*, I reminded myself. *You are a mourner. Act like a mourner.*

The funeral director appeared at my elbow, her hands demurely clasped. Did I want to do an identification?

It sounded so *CSI* that I nearly laughed. They hadn't pulled her body out of a river, or out of the rafters of an abandoned warehouse with a gunshot wound in the back of the head. They'd taken her from a hospital morgue, wearing a bracelet with her name on it. Who else could it be? I stopped myself: This was my mother we were talking about. The body in the coffin could be anyone. *She* could be anywhere.

"Do I want to see her?" I said to Arie under my breath. I had only ever seen one dead body, an over-rouged, plasticky mannequin at a Catholic wake. I didn't want to sear a traumatic memory into my mind. But neither would I ever, otherwise, be sure it was her. She'd pulled off crazier stunts. This was a woman who'd given birth to me at home in the 70s with the aid of an unlicensed midwife; who'd bribed the super to drill a hole in the wall between her bedroom and the living room so she could keep the oxygen tank in one room and puff away on her cigarette with equanimity in the other; who'd lied with a perfectly straight face about such small matters as the identity of my father, her real last name, the number of times she'd been married, my Social Security number. Only a fool would have put faking her own death beyond her.

Arie hesitated. "It would give you a chance to say anything to her that you didn't get a chance to say when she was alive. And we could be sure she . . . looks okay," he said carefully.

I dispatched the funeral director, who opened the back of the hearse and slid aside the top of the coffin, peering in. She stepped back and nodded. I clutched Arie's suited arm, and we moved around the back of the car. I stepped around the open door.

Jews: let me give you the warning I didn't get.

As requested, she was in the traditional shroud. A shroud, it turns out, is not a mummy-style sheet. It's a kittel, a ritual garment like an ankle-length button-down shirt, tied at the waist.

And it comes with—get this—a matching bonnet. Frilled around the face, tied in a neat bow under the chin. God help me, my first thought was: *That's not my mother. It's the ghost of Laura Ingalls Wilder.*

I had always hung onto the idea that I could only believe the things about my mother that I could see with my own eyes. And here she was.

She looked more peaceful than she ever had in life. I'm sure the funeral home sewed her mouth and eyelids shut, and put some blush on; regardless, she looked not just asleep but like she was having a calm and happy dream. She had lost a lot of weight once her dentures stopped fitting well, and her face was narrower than I remembered it. I smoothed the coarse gray hair trailing out from the bonnet and touched her forehead; her skin was fridge cold and dense, like a block of fresh mozzarella. My finger burned for hours, until I finally ran it under the hottest water I could stand.

I told her I loved her. I told her I was sorry I wasn't with her when she died, and that I hadn't told her then. That I was sorry she had such a hard life. That I forgave her, and that I was sorry too. That I hoped she was at peace, and that she and Ruth were together. I told her goodbye.

When I stepped away, the funeral director handed me an envelope. "This is all we got from the hospital," she said.

I opened it and shook a cheap black Casio watch into my

hand. "No clothes or anything?" I asked. "Presumably she didn't go to the hospital naked. I mean. I assume. I wouldn't actually put it past her."

Arie squeezed my arm, and the funeral director smiled gently; uncomfortable, verge-of-tears jokes must have been familiar to her. "Nothing else," she said.

I opened my mouth with another poor attempt at humor— something like Lady Godiva, Zombie Edition—and was thankfully interrupted by the arrival of the eight months pregnant rabbi, who heaved herself out of an Uber, resplendent in a rainbow kippah. *Mom would've loved this*, I thought. She hugged me fiercely, twisting her body to keep her belly out of the way. The cantor produced a sheaf of handouts. The funeral director closed the casket. We were ready.

Standing off to the side of our now-silent friends, we performed the keriah, the rending ceremony, and pinned the torn black ribbon to our clothes. The rabbi took me by the elbow and looked into my eyes.

"God has given," she said.

"*God has given,*" we repeated.

"God has taken."

"*God has taken.*"

She steadied my arm.

"Blessed be God's name."

We piled into the cars and drove slowly up a bumpy dirt road in the crowded cemetery, the shoulders of gravestones jostling each other for space. The gravediggers shifted the coffin to a wheeled dolly and wound it deftly through the thicket to the open grave, the raw, orange earth crumbling to the side. I scraped my shin on a child's duckling-topped gravestone, and absentmindedly apologized to it. We gathered silently in an uneven circle.

"Thank you for gathering here with us this morning," the rabbi began. "We come together today to honor the life of Judith Scheier. Jewish tradition marks for us a time to begin coming to terms with a world that has been altered—for some just a little and for others immensely—by the loss of her soul. We name with honesty the fact that Judith"—*Not her first name! She'll eat you alive!* I thought wildly, automatically—"always tried her best throughout her life, and with equal honesty we reflect that sometimes her best was not enough for what her life demanded. But Judaism also teaches that the world would not be the same without her presence, and we know that the world will not be the same in her absence."

Rachel escaped from her grandparents and ran to the center of the circle, spinning gleefully. She noticed the coffin and stopped, toe in the dust, considering. "Daddy!" she called, pointing. "Someone isn't here. Someone isn't here!" Everyone shifted uncomfortably. *Great*, I thought. *My daughter is a witch.*

We recited the psalms. Psalms 121—*I lift up my eyes to the hills, where does my help come from?*—and 23—*Adonai is my shepherd; I shall not want.* The cantor sang "El Malei Rachamim"—*Compassionate God, Eternal Spirit of the universe, grant perfect rest in your sheltering presence to Judith Scheier-Tzena Feyge bat Louis v'Ruth, who has entered eternity. Source of mercy, let her find refuge in the shadow of your wings, and let her soul be bound up in the bond of everlasting life. God is her inheritance. May she rest in peace, and let us say: amen.* My non-Jewish friends stumbled over the words, but kept going gamely.

A loud knock came from the grave, and those closest to it

jumped. *Here we go,* I thought. *If anyone was going to* Goonies *her own burial, it's Mom.* Probably a clump of earth falling. Probably a loose stone hitting wood. Probably.

The burial team were dressed to match the raw earth, orange and brown, with broad-brimmed floppy hats and bandanas over their noses. They lowered the coffin off the dolly onto the wood supports, ran long straps underneath it, and on a silent count, pulled out the supports and lowered the coffin into the grave. I expected this to be the worst moment. I had braced for it. But all I felt was a cold, full-body wash of relief. It felt like putting my frazzled cat back into the carrier after a vet appointment, like lowering my flushed toddler, overtired and weeping, into her crib. It felt like stepping painfully into the hotel shower after the marathon, my muscles unhitching under the steaming water. Like scrunching down under a cool sheet, flushed scarlet with the flu. The relief, the exhale, the curl—finally—into the small and safe place. It's an old, crowded cemetery, and her barely cold body could not have been more than a foot from her mother's skeleton. This space in the earth, hacked out and sun warmed, had been waiting for her for the sixty years since she had stood and watched Ruth lowered into it. She had prayed every day to get there. Now there she was, lying flat in a thin pine box topped with a skinny wooden Star of David, arms at her side and incongruous bow knotted carefully under her chin. She was finally home.

The rabbi gave directions, softly. We were to step up, take the shovel out of the earth, dump in a scoop of dirt, and stab the shovel back in. There would be no passing the shovel from hand to hand. No shortcuts. Often, she said gently, mourners use the back of the shovel to pass the earth, demonstrating a reluctance, a protest that their loved one was gone. She gestured to me. Ready.

I stepped forward and Excalibured the heavy shovel out of the ground, my heels sinking alarmingly. I flipped the shovel right side up. I scooped up the dirt, and I dropped it into the grave. Arie followed me, his eyes downcast. One by one, my friends picked their way across the crumbling earth and dropped in their own shovelfuls, burying her with me.

The rabbi stepped forward and took the shovel. Maneuvering her arms past her belly, she scattered earth lightly over the coffin so that the lid was obscured. Her methodical movements reminded me exactly of myself smoothing a sheet over one of the kids' mattresses. I couldn't help feeling like we were tucking her in.

We said Kaddish, and sang the *oseh shalom*. And that was it. We looked around at each other, and then fell into an awkward line back to the path. We hugged, one at a time, and people trailed off to return to their regular lives—Gabriela to catch a plane; Tor's wife to drive her weeping husband home; Carol to return to Connecticut, silent, her oldest friend dead and buried. As we walked away, the burial team was already filling in the grave with fast, practiced movements, eager to get out of the sun.

Under normal circumstances, you'd go back to the deceased's house to sit shiva. You'd sit on a low chair and eat platters of food brought by your friends and family and you'd let yourself wallow. You'd be *required* to wallow. Jewish culture is antithetical to so much about American life, and the strictly mandated periods of work and rest, feast and fast, holiday and weekday, the period of mourning and the days after, speak to an understanding the secular world lacks, that the soul moves on its own time. A mourner is not expected to say goodbye, bury their dead, and show up at work the next morning with hair neatly combed. Tradition dictates that while the burial is for the deceased, the shiva is for those left behind. Front doors are left unlocked and guests enter without ringing the bell, quietly, gauging the tenor of the room before they speak. If the mourner is weeping, they offer hugs but don't make a show of greeting them. If the mourner is laughing and telling stories, they listen and laugh with them. There is no pressure to pretend you're OK when you're definitely not OK.

Under normal circumstances, I would have waded into the piles of paperwork, liquidated her accounts, and managed her will. There would have been conflict with family members about who got which ugly cocktail ring, who kept which photo. Someone would have broken down crying as we sorted through her clothing.

But these were not normal circumstances. The apartment in which we should have held a shiva was even now being renovated for a new, full rent–paying tenant. She died with only a few bills in her wallet, and six figures of debt to the landlord. And there was no one else left to mourn her. I stood next to the car with my squirming son in my arms, thinking, with some dread: *When will people expect me to be normal? When the meals stop coming, when the sympathy cards stop arriving, when I start counting her absence in weeks and months and not in hours— when do I have to be a person again?*

My daughter spun around my husband, singing tunelessly to herself, and the heat of the sun beat down. The rabbi and the cantor juggled their bags, packing away the leftover handouts. Car doors slammed shut down the path. I got in the car and we drove away, the children shrieking gleefully in their car seats and the white glare of the sun over everything.

✦ ✦ ✦

The rabbi had gotten across, succinctly, everything I had said to her the night my mother died. She had tried her best, but because of her hard life, and because of her illness, her best had not been enough. I wanted to get across that two opposing things can be true. She was a chaos monger, and she had brought much of this trouble on herself, and also she was a sick, vulnerable old woman to whom terrible things happened in the last few months of her life. It's easy to think of reaction to abuse as a binary: you're under the abuser's thumb, or you've cut them off. But that's not always how it goes. You can still love someone who has caused you a lot of harm. You can want to protect them from some of the shittier things the world throws at them. It is really, really hard to know where the line between enabling and rescuing is, especially when mental illness is at play. Friends from normal families would shake their heads when I told them about her worse days and ask why I didn't just cut her off, that she would fend for herself, that I was being codependent.

Maybe I was. But it wasn't so easy for me to know where to draw that line. She shrieked at me hysterically on the phone for hours on end *and also* she didn't have money for rent; she lied about who my father was *and also* she was in pain, physical and psychic, every day of her life.

Now that I have my own children, I see how much of her best my mother did. She tried. She gave me what she could, and she protected me from everything she could, and she loved me with all her heart. But love doesn't solve everything. It isn't even always a net positive. Love is like alcohol: it takes what you are and exacerbates it. If you live from crisis to crisis and from anger to fury, that's what your love tastes like.

But: she tried.

I thought about that service a lot in the days after the burial. Organized religion takes a lot of guff for being, well, organized. The standard prayers, repeated verbatim, are criticized for being rote and irrelevant. But I found the lack of personalization very comforting. The service is all about God, and assumes nothing about the people reciting the prayers, or about their relationship to the deceased. As she had instructed, I didn't give a eulogy, and no one expected me to cry, although I did.

The burial service acknowledges the passing and the change of death without any sop about the perfection of the mother-daughter bond or the perfection of the deceased. These words had been recited by millions before me, said with love and with anger and with grief and with weariness and with indifference. They assume nothing. They leave room to grieve a person and grieve a relationship, separately. I, Nechama Gila, daughter of Tzena Fayge, put my mother in the ground. Not her beloved or loving daughter, not her unconflicted, adoring, or mourning daughter. But she had conceived me and carried me and gave birth to me, sweating and screaming, sixteen floors above First Avenue. Say what you will about the rigidity of tradition, but it gave me a framework to work from when I had no idea what to do or how to feel.

❖ ❖ ❖

We drove back through Brooklyn and stopped at Mermaid Manor to see if we could pick up my mother's belongings. Arie stayed in the car and plied the kids with crackers. Elderly people lined the outside of the building, standing or seated on those walkers with seats. They were mostly men. I couldn't make the automatic doors open, and a grinning character in a tan newsboy cap pointed me to the handicap button. I made it through the doors and felt their eyes on my ass in my tall heels and black dress; in a new sedate city and with two small children tagging my feet, street harassment was a thing of distant memory, and the annoyance almost made me feel nostalgic.

The lobby looked like a doctor's waiting room, with long banks of plastic seating. Nearly every chair was full. It smelled good, clean. Most people chatted with their neighbor, or listened contentedly to portable CD players. A man dropped his cane, which clattered to the floor; he caught my arm as he went down and I pulled him back up to standing.

A polite receptionist took my name and made a hushed call: "the daughter" was here. I was awash in relief. I had expected something like the SROs I'd visited in my work with the Coalition for the Homeless, roach infested and full of residents who were getting none of the care they needed. This place was bland but serviceable.

Irina the social worker was younger than I expected, a warm, padded woman who talked at a pell-mell, rapid pace. God, I missed Queens. We walked up the stairs to Mom's locked bedroom.

She had taken a giant, ancient suitcase to the shelter, a black-and-yellow number from the days before wheeled rollaboards. It weighed a ton, and I wrestled it down the elevator and out of the building while silent care workers stared after me and Irina called: "I am so sorry! I don't know what hap-pened with her! You look beautiful!" Arie hoisted it into the trunk, and we left Brooklyn with my mother's last belongings riding silently behind us.

I opened it that night, thinking: *Get this over with.* It smelled like her, a mix of Emeraude, Dove soap, and cigarettes. I lost it then. I love smells; if I've been to your house and gone to your bathroom, I've smelled your conditioner. This scent was par-ticular to her skin, that cold skin we had put into the ground only hours before to bloat, leak, and rot. When this scent wore off there would be no more.

There were clothes, nothing I recognized. Clean, medical-looking bras. Black T-shirts from the shelter. A baggie full of her and her mother's costume jewelry, much to the credit of the ALF staff; I thought of the suitcase sitting silently unattended in her room while she raged in the hospital, then being neatly packed by an indifferent care worker. A rubber foot scrubber. A travel comb with her hair still tangled in it. The scroll from her mezuzah; I pictured her stopping the marshal from clos-ing the door so she could reach up with shaking fingers and pull it out. A toothbrush still crusted with toothpaste crud. A Hershey's bar, and three packs of cinnamon gum. Baby wipes. My old point-and-shoot camera bag, empty. A small notebook in which she'd kept track of birthdays and anniversaries. Her birth certificate, a hand-filled-out form that looked comically old-fashioned. A bunch of keys. A clean but badly torn night-gown. (Who had done her laundry in the shelter? Or did she just not change?) Two rolls of toilet paper.

Yumi had gone to the hospital's security room, notarized release form in hand, to pick up her possessions. I'd promised to send FedEx to do a pickup if she had anything heavy, but that was a hilariously bad assumption. She had taken nothing to the hospital but her wallet and her keys, keys that opened a door to a home that was no longer hers.

Her wallet was a portable parody of a competent adult's. Her driver's license had expired; she carried a debit card from a bank where she hadn't had an account in fifteen years. Maybe she'd just forgotten to clean it out. Or maybe she was putting on a show of a person who had a bank account, who hadn't picked a fight with so many tellers that she ended up shutting down her accounts out of righteous pride. She was playing the role of a normal person until the very end.

In Jewish tradition, the soul hovers near the body for three days, confused, before it departs our world. It's a mitzvah to perform a *shemira* call, derived from the words for "watching" or "guardian"; the person sits in the room with the body, or outside the refrigerator if the burial has been delayed, reading psalms. I did this once for a longtime congregant of my synagogue, during the four a.m. to six a.m. shift. If you're wondering: yes, a funeral home is fucking creepy before dawn. A friend came to relieve me at six, and I about climbed him like a tree. I wondered if there was some of my mother still clinging to this small, prosaic pile of belongings.

Over the next week, I looked up forensics sites, past caring what my company's IT team might think of my browsing history. I found myself poring for hours over websites that detailed the process of human decomposition. I wanted to know what was happening to her body. I was fascinated, and surprisingly untroubled by the (literally) gory details. When would her cheeks fall in? When would the flesh rot away? What was left in Ruth's sixty-year-old grave next door—what had welcomed her when they lowered her into the ground? I knew when she would turn from green to red, when mold would grow on her cheeks, when the gases would release. I knew that in a month—especially in a stifling New York August—she would be mostly skeleton and liquid. I found it all both horrifying and comforting. The earth was taking her back. She was, after all that, only human, imperfect and formed out of soft tissue. Her rage was not embalming fluid. She could not escape the universal end.

The internet is full of pictures of decomposing bodies—do *not* google this unless you are very much sure you want to—too often with disconcertingly bound hands, or curled sleeplike into soaked-through beds. I thought of Bridget Jones, fearful that her spinster corpse would be found a week later, half-eaten by Alsatians, and was grateful that my mother had died with someone, even strangers, by her side.

Most non-Orthodox Jews don't have much interest in the afterlife. We have no concept of personal salvation, and are murky on the concept of divine rewards or punishments. I don't know where my mother is now. I can't say that I would want to be reunited with her as she was later in life; the image of us perched on the clouds somewhere, arguing at the top of our trumpet-peal voices, is appealing for comedy's sake but also ridiculous. It's comforting to think that she and Ruth are back together, and that they are being kinder to each other reunited than they were in life. But I know that what she really wanted was an end. She was exhausted. She was ready to leave behind the body that was failing her, the mind that sent up signal flares she couldn't predict or control, and a world she found increasingly bizarre and hard to navigate.

The world without her felt safer than it ever had before. Life is bonkers and any given day might bring *some* kind of chaos, but it was no longer likely it was *her* kind of chaos. Maybe she'd booby-trapped something. Maybe there were more lawyers and surprises and madness yet to come. But there was now an immovable stopping point. This would not, after all, spin out forever.

Ask me again in the years to come and I may feel differently, but in this immediate aftermath I am finding my mother much easier to love as an icon and as a series of great and funny stories than I did as a person. She had many good qualities, and, as Arie pointed out, she was both dealt a bad hand and played that hand badly. I hope that I can let the good stories surface and the bad ones sink for good. I hope I can remember her as she would have liked to be remembered: flawed, but well-intentioned.

A very wise friend pointed out that this kind of grief hits in strange ways, because the sudden relief from the daily crises and the worry about what-the-hell-this-time every time the phone rings leaves me with a known entity to mourn. For the first time, I can think of her as a person and not as a badly wound alarm clock, shrieking at random, startling the birds.

I didn't mourn my mother's existence. In her last few years, she was not a part of my daily life. I didn't mourn heart-to-heart conversations that didn't occur, or a loving relationship that just wasn't. I mourned the closing of a door that couldn't reopen. Lies can be corrected and the truth told. When the truth-holder loses her memory there is still hope: memories still surface and loom, summoned by a word here and an image there. But with that last electrical current flickered out, her lips stitched shut and her tongue collapsed forever, there was no one left to tell her stories, true or not.

This is a function of old age and isolation. Warren's sister Helen must remember a lot of what he did. They grew up in the same house, knew the same parents, saw the same things. It's said that siblings grow up with different parents, but some of the major events of their childhood—the crane-hoisted toy giraffe, the unconscious mother sprawled on the living room floor—they would both remember. For all my life I mistrusted my own memory and wished for an independent witness to confirm: yes, she said this; yes, you screamed that; yes, that happened. A sibling would have been useful for this, or a father. To this day differing memories terrify me, even totally inconsequential ones—"No," my husband will say offhandedly, "you didn't want the birthday party to start at three, I did," and my brain spins off frantically. Did I? Did he? Can my memory be trusted? Will I ever know what really happened?

I grieved, but for the first time in my life my heart didn't sink when the phone rang. The last few years had been so chaotic, so filled with surprises and mysteries. A constant loop of making decisions with partial information and of reviewing every statement. Every day I hashed and rehashed the question of one person's responsibility to another. I was finally relieved of the constant worry about whether I could make better decisions about my mother's life than she could; she lied so thoroughly and so often that I always second-guessed myself, knowing she could well know something I didn't. It turns out that she didn't.

It's hard to comprehend a world without my mother in it. My mother, the panopticon personified: who threatened to remove my door from its hinges if I closed it, who read my letters and asked my teachers to track my movements, who threatened to hire college students to follow me on the street. When she wasn't there in person she called, many times a day. She got my aunt to print and send her all the pictures from my Facebook page, which she pinned haphazardly to a wall like a TV detective sorting through a list of suspects. I carved out mind space that was safe and separate from her, but a space formed in reaction to someone has the outline of that person in it.

Grief didn't feel like the wolf gnawing at my innards. There was no shaking, no weeping. I wasn't in a fetal position with the covers over my head. It felt like a diving belt, keeping me just below the surface and just below normal. I went to work and to the gym. I sat on the Metro and shopped for groceries. And every place I went, my eyes were filmy and damp. I wish I had had the breakdown instead, some dramatic blowup from which I could have recovered, instead of this grayed-out sadness.

On the morning of her shiva service, it was a blistering ninety degrees by ten a.m. I showered off the DC sweat and on a whim, put on the only unripped housedress I'd found in her luggage from the shelter—a midcalf-length, flutter-sleeved black smock printed with tropical fruit. And pockets! *Pockets.* She had left me a perfect garment. I swanned around the house humming, tidying up clutter and spot-cleaning, and suddenly the doorbell rang; I opened it, expecting another delivery of flowers or a condolence fruit basket, and there stood my most stylish acquaintance, a pixie-haired beauty who looked fresh and perfect even though she was hugely pregnant and it was furnace-hot out. I accepted the giant bag of shiva food and prepared dinners she handed me, and tried not to cry—both from sheer emotion from her kindness, and from the exhausted knowledge that I'd just faced down Glory while wearing a muumuu.

At the shiva service, my living room filled with the motley mix of friends we'd made or kept in DC—some friends from college, friends from synagogue, members of my book club, Laura's wonderful uncle whom I'd secretly always hoped liked me better—I put out an assortment of the food people had sent, and on impulse stuck a late 60s–era picture of her in a frame and propped it up among the plates. No coy wedding photo or friendly family reunion shot for her shiva. In it, she wears a long-sleeved purple minidress ("I showed off the legs because I didn't have the boobs, honey!") and her strawberry-blond hair is blown into a perfect, smooth flip. She pouts up at the camera. Given the date, it must have been taken by her first husband. This is a Judith Scheier I never knew—sexy, playful, glamorous. Guests glanced at it while reaching for the onion dip, did a double take, looked again, glanced at me. I smiled, showing all my teeth.

A month after she died, I called her number from an airport gate. I wouldn't have been surprised if she'd picked up. This was the woman who'd raised me in one of the most expensive cities in the world on zero income, who chain-smoked while wearing an oxygen mask, who maintained perfectly separate lives and elaborate lies for decades. Surely a phone call from beyond the grave was within her means. She loved that phone number; she'd bullied a representative from Ma Bell and then AT&T into granting her a number ending in two zeros, businesslike and easy to remember.

The phone rang, hollow in my ear, and I tried to think of what I'd say if the number had already been reassigned and the poor unfortunate soul picked up. But the innocents of the 212 area code were spared from me that day. It rang and rang, and eventually I ended the call, side-eyeing other travelers to see if they could tell that I was clearly having a breakdown of some kind.

From then on I did most of my crying at the gym. I went to an absurdly titled high-rep weights class ("Body Pump," if you must know; I know, I *know*) that always ended with power ballads, and I sang along to them as I crunched my core in ridiculous positions, swabbing at my cheeks when they were wet. Then, in the institutional shower, I stood under luke-warm water and sobbed some more, confident no one would hear me. I missed New York, where you could cry in public— Didn't *How I Met Your Mother* even have a running gag about this?—without being bothered, or only by a good-natured older woman who'd pass you a tissue and pat you too hard on the back. DC is so cold, so stiff upper lip, so WASP-y; no mat-ter what's going on; you're fine in public, FINE. I wasn't fine.

✦ ✦ ✦

The friend who'd told me I wasn't too special to have children came to my rescue with a view of the future I could live with. "Your kids will only know her through your eyes," she said. "You can tell her story differently. You can cast her mental illness as eccentricity, her inconsistency as zaniness. And in time it will become true. The edges will smooth out. Charac-ter will become caricature. She'll be a story, not a weapon." *Yes,* I thought. *I can remake these stories to make her sound like Auntie Mame with a raucous, smoke-infused Queens accent, rather than a gorgon who turned her every fear into a wall around me.*

My kids are too young to ask about my mother, or about Warren. They don't really understand that their beloved Mar-tin and Bibi, for whom they dance and ham it up over video chat several times a week, are their father's own parents; in their eyes we're all just *there*, like mountains, or newspapers, or coffee mugs. In their minds, the only important people are the ones they see in front of them. And that's just fine.

What will I tell them when they're old enough? Probably

nothing. I'll read them her ancient, annotated *Winnie-the-Pooh* in which all the characters are female. I'll sing them "A Bushel and a Peck" in the bathtub, like she did, enthusiastically and tunelessly, for me. I'll buy them ice cream on the first day of school to remind them that learning is sweet. And of our shared history, I'll give them the sanitized version: Your grandfather was sick when he was young, and then he died. Your grandmother was young and sick, and then she had me, and over time she got old and sick, and then she died. I don't want to weigh them down with the empty hole of a missing parent, the inconsolable grief I've been kicking down the years. I don't want them to know that parents can be as dangerous as they can be loving. Arie and I aren't perfect, of course, and neither are our kids. I've got years of grounding them ahead of me. Phones to take away. Friends to disapprove of. There are endless ways to fuck up as a parent. I want them to think that my ways are the worst it gets.

Maybe when they're older, and they start to see me and their father as real people with separate thoughts and separate lives. Maybe then I'll give them a truncated version of the truth. They don't need the ugly details. I'll leave out the crack of my skull against the doorframe, and the middle-of-the-night photo-ripping frenzy, and the haze of adrenaline in the air when rage filled my mother's body like oil fills a jar.

I will tell them the good stories and leave out the bad. I'll tell them the time-softened truth. I'll tell them the legend that is based in indisputable reality. I'll tell them what I know for sure to be real. That Judith Scheier loved me, and that she did the best she could.

Because when it comes to love, I'm a liar too.

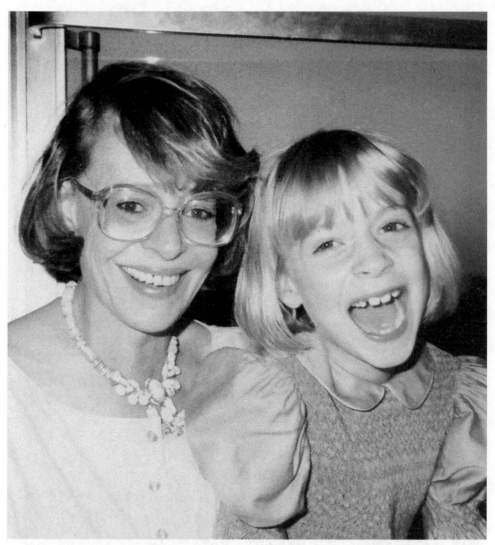

Me with my mother around 1986. I inherited her penchant for bangs, but not, apparently, her poise.

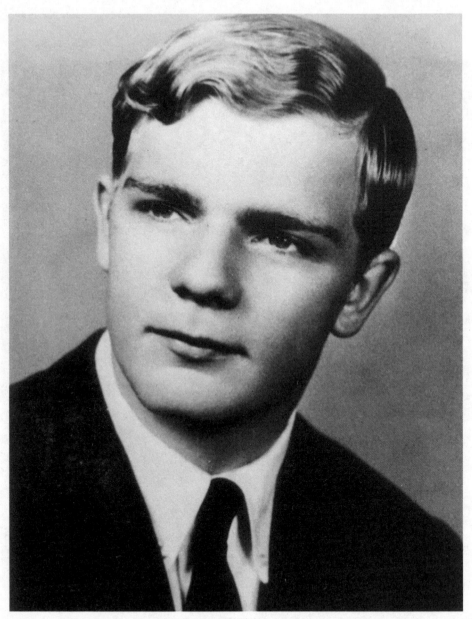

Warren Luther's 1967 photo in The Dutchman, *Collegiate's yearbook*

Acknowledgments

For the first full year, I didn't tell anyone I was writing this book. Instead I spent my lunch hour hiding in the corner of the staff lounge, typing madly away, turning a rabid-dog eye on anyone who approached and growling softly in warning, half a sandwich trembling in my jaws.

Looking back, that was a colossally dumb move. Do you know how nice people are to you when you admit you're writing a book, even though you have zero (ZERO) idea what you're doing? SO NICE.

I owe a debt of gratitude to so many people. Let it be known that this is a woefully incomplete list.

Alexa Zimmerman, Gabriela Allen, Jess Rogers, Marie-Amélie George, Molly Pachence, and Yumi Kim. No human being on earth has ever before been so lucky as to have such an amazing pit crew stick by her decade after decade. Thank you from the stringy, cantankerous depths of my heart.

Claire Whitman and Caitlin Nye, without whose fine-upstanding-human-being example, encouragement, good humor, and sly wit I would have trebucheted this manuscript into a ditch a long time ago.

Kez Quin, Libby Mosier, and Rachel Simon, writing teachers who became beloved friends, for which I am forever grateful.

Rabbis Sharon Kleinbaum, Rachel Weiss, and Yael Rapport for guidance both spiritual and pragmatic.

Julia Dunkin, Roslyn Deasing, Madeline Santiago, Nichole Reid, Jessica Mendez, and all the other women who cared for my mother even when she screamed, swore, threw things, and called you names. You have my profound respect and gratitude. Thank you.

Michele Rubin, who gave critical early feedback.

Serena Jones, whose thoughtful comments and wry, heartfelt humor were a ballast when I was floundering around in a sea of my own overwrought adjectives. Thank you for taking a chance on me.

Team Holt: Amy Einhorn for taking a flyer on a total unknown, Anita Sheih and Hannah Campbell for keeping everything running smoothly, Janel Brown and Amy Medeiros for their keen eyes, which saved me from humiliating myself (too much), and Jason Liebman, Callum Plews, Meryl Sussman Levavi, Marian Brown, Maia Sacca-Schaeffer, Allison Carney, Jaya Miceli, and Chris Sergio for your hard work and guidance in getting this story from manuscript to book. Thank you, thank you, thank you.

Christopher Schelling, possessor of the World's Best Laugh™, whose skills at agenting are superseded only by his innate talent for friendship. For both of these I am eternally grateful.

And finally: my brilliant, hilarious, endlessly entertaining husband, Arie, without whom no story would have as much savor and no memory as much joy. I love you, Best Person.

About the Author

Liz Scheier is a product developer living in Washington, DC, with her husband, two small children, and an ill-behaved cat. This is her first book. She is working on the second.